Sexual Pleasure

No matter what your level of experience or satisfaction with your sex life, you can benefit from the increased sense of playfulness and deeper sensual enjoyment that the ideas in *Sexual Pleasure* will add to your lovemaking. By following the exercises and focusing on what truly pleases *you*, you and your lover will discover a new world of wondrous and revitalized sex.

Sexual Pleasure will teach you:

- simple body image work and self-caress techniques to lay the foundation for profound sensual awareness

- the essential differences between female and male arousal, and how they can complement each other for maximum pleasure

- how to focus attention at the exact point of touch—whether you are touching or being touched—which makes you forget your anxieties and reduces performance pressure

- how to last longer: exercises to intensify your arousal and prolong sexual pleasure

- ways to build trust, enhance intimacy, and heighten the desire between you and your partner

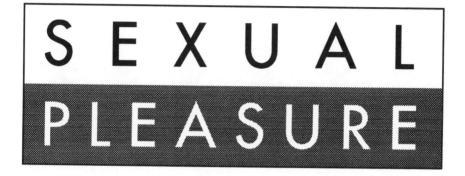

SEXUAL PLEASURE

Reaching New Heights
of Sexual Arousal
& Intimacy

Barbara Keesling, Ph.D.

Hunter
House

Photographs reprinted from *Erotic by Nature: A Celebration of Life, of Love, and of Our Wonderful Bodies*, David Steinberg, ed., Down There Press/Red Alder Books, 1988. © 1988 by David Steinberg. Reprinted by permission.

Illustrations in Appendix A reprinted from *The Fertility Awareness Handbook* © 1981 Barbara Kass-Annese and Hal Danzer, Hunter House Inc., Publishers 1992. Reprinted by permission.

Library of Congress Cataloging-in-Publication Data

Keesling, Barbara.
Sexual pleasure : reaching new heights of sexual arousal and intimacy /
Barbara Keesling.
p. cm.   Includes index.
ISBN 0-89793-149-1 : $21.95 — ISBN 0-89793-148-3 (pbk.) : $12.95
1. Sex instruction 2. Sex (Psychology) I. Title.
HQ31.K393 1993
613.9'6—dc20   93-23625

ORDERING: *Trade bookstores and wholesalers in the U.S. and Canada, please contact:*
Publishers Group West
4065 Hollis Street, Box 8843
Emeryville CA 94608   Phone: (800) 788-3123   Fax: (510) 658-1834

Special sales: Hunter House books are available at special discounts for sales promotions, organizations, premiums, fundraising, and for educational use.
For details please contact:

Special Sales Department
Hunter House Inc., Publishers
P.O. Box 2914
Alameda CA 94501-0914   Phone: (510) 865-5282   Fax: (510) 865-4295

Cover Design: Timm Sinclair and Jil Weil   Book design: *Qalagraphia*
Project Editor: Lisa E. Lee   Editor: Deborah A. Grandinetti
Production Manager: Paul J. Frindt
Marketing: Corrine M. Sahli   Promotion: Robin Donovan
Customer Service: Laura O'Brien   Fulfillment: Sergio Gaspari
Publisher: Kiran S. Rana
Printed and bound by Publishers Press, Salt Lake City UT
Manufactured in the United States of America

First edition

Contents

Exercises and
Bonding Explorations

Exercises

Acknowledgments

I would like to thank all of the people who helped with this book. Many of the exercises described in *Sexual Pleasure* were taught to me by Michael Riskin, Anita Banker, and Ron Gibb.

I would like to thank Kiran Rana and the staff at Hunter House, including Paul, Lisa, Robin, Corrie, and Laura. I would also like to thank Deborah Grandinetti and Jackie Melvin for their editorial work.

I would also like to thank my husband, John, for his emotional support and for helping me with word processing.

This book is dedicated to my clients

Introduction

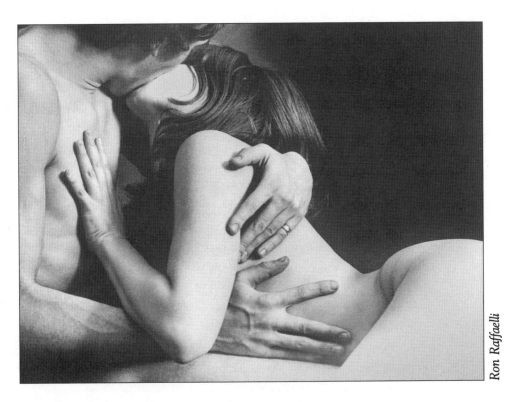

Ron Raffaelli

Making Love Better Than Ever

This is a book about how to fall in love—together—with the pleasures of the body.

It is about *coming home* to what pleases *you* and achieving the mastery over your body that will take your lovemaking to new heights. It is about letting go of agendas, or trying to "turn on" your partner. It is about unlearning all of the attitudes that keep you from fully enjoying yourself, and each other.

Sexual Pleasure's philosophy is quite controversial in this regard. Yet it has been proven repeatedly by many sex therapists and researchers. The philosophy is this: by learning to focus on your own sensations and enjoyment, you will actually become *more* sensitive to your partner's feelings and needs. Discovering what you enjoy can build your confidence, make it easier to ask for what you want, and bring a new sense of freedom in bed.

Many other sexual advice books emphasize the need to please your partner at the expense of pleasing yourself. Credentialed therapists and self-styled experts alike may peddle this approach. I think it's harmful. I have seen it lead to performance anxiety. I have seen it alienate lovers who are simply trying to get closer.

Let me tell you what else doesn't work. I do not believe in

the "try this position" or "try this technique," cookbook approach to sex. Developing your lovemaking to the point where it is as pleasurable and mutually satisfying as possible takes more than a positive attitude, an erotic setting, or a specific technique. The real secret is in developing *sensuality*—an appreciation for the many nuances of feeling and the exquisite range of sensation of which the body is capable. The only real essentials of sexual pleasure, which you can develop with experience and practice, are:

- fully *enjoying touching*, your partner or yourself

- fully *enjoying being touched*, by your partner or yourself

- fully *enjoying yourself* during lovemaking, without anxiety or guilt

With these three basics, touch and feeling merge as a medium of experience and expression, and lovemaking becomes a deeply physical and emotional exchange that revitalizes and sustains you at all levels of being.

Isn't this refreshingly simple?

Sexual Pleasure will help you develop this sensual awareness, through exercises that increase sexual desire, deepen arousal, and enhance intimacy. I have carefully arranged these exercises in a graduated program. They range from simple self-caress techniques that can be practiced alone to partner exercises that allow you reach intense levels of arousal and sustained orgasm. These latter exercises are best enjoyed in a strong, intimate relationship in which you share great emotional trust.

These exercises are known to sex therapists as "sensate focus exercises." They represent a refinement of an approach pioneered by the well-known sex therapists William Masters and Virginia Johnson.

Masters and Johnson devised these behavioral exercises back in the 1950s and 1960s to help people effectively overcome sexual problems. But their usefulness does not stop there. I've found that sensate focus can have even more to offer couples who have no real problems to speak of, but who are looking for a way to make love better than ever. It is for couples like these that I have written *Sexual Pleasure*.

Many of the exercises in this book are new and are being published for the first time. They are not even widely known among most therapists. In fact, when my colleagues and I speak at professional conferences, we find that the great majority of general therapists are unfamiliar with any sex therapy techniques except for the "squeeze" technique and the "stop-start" technique (both of which are for premature ejaculation). In just this one book, I will give you more than *fifty* exercises!

All of the exercises in *Sexual Pleasure* make use of the very latest research. The ones I have included on arousal, for instance, are based on current findings about male and female arousal patterns. They build on the Masters and Johnson sensate focus approach, but go much farther.

My colleagues and I have developed some of these techniques together. My own contribution has been to take sensate focus and make it much more sexual. Among the exercises you won't find elsewhere are ones that tell how to:

- increase staying power for both men and women

- have more control over erections

- make ejaculation more enjoyable

- help women reach orgasm readily

Who Can Use This Book?

With the techniques and approaches given in this book, anyone at any age or experience level can get more out of sex than they currently do. The exercises described in *Sexual Pleasure* can be used by anyone who would like to increase their sexual desire, deepen arousal, strengthen orgasm, and enhance intimacy in their relationship.

While I have written this book with heterosexual couples in mind, many of these exercises can be used by same sex couples, since the sensate focus process is enriching for everybody. You can even start this program if you have no sexual experience at all. You will also find them helpful if you have a specific sexual problem, such as difficulty keeping erections or experiencing orgasms.

The exercises can be adapted for use by people who have physical limitations due to illness or age. They are not strenuous. If you have arthritis or knee problems, it may help to do the intercourse exercises in a side-to-side position rather than with one partner on top. If you have a heart condition, however, please check with your doctor before starting on this, or any program of increased physical activity.

If you are a male or female survivor of sexual abuse, you may find that reading this book brings back many painful memories. If you do want to learn this material, however, consider working through it with a therapist's guidance. Experiencing these exercises with a loving, supportive partner can bring real healing, but it will take time and require you to develop enough trust so that you feel safe with your lover.

Whether you are an abuse survivor or not, you need to be aware that the intimate touch in these exercises will stir emotions. Sharing profound sensual and sexual pleasure awakens deeper aspects of ourselves. This can be wonderful and empowering, but if the intimate work raises issues that become too challenging for you, please stop the exercises and seek the help of a professional counselor.

Because of the emotional impact of these exercises, I recommend them most for couples who are willing to develop the patience, commitment, honesty, and openness that is the foundation of a strong relationship. Changing the way you make love can also change you and your relationship. It is important for each of you to be aware of this.

What You'll Find in Sexual Pleasure

Sexual Pleasure is divided into four sections—Sensational Sexuality, Sexual Arousal and Men, Sexual Arousal and Women, and Mutuality and Intimacy. Sensational Sexuality (Part I) contains chapters on how to touch and how to relax. This is basic information about your body that you should know before you begin any touching exercises. Part I also contains exercises that you can do by yourself to explore and get to know your own sexual responses. Finally, Part I contains a chapter on increasing sexual desire through sensual exercises with your partner. The chapters in Part I give you the foundation for the more advanced exercises that follow in Parts II, III, and IV.

Sexual Arousal and Men (Part II) includes four chapters. The first is on male sexual response. This chapter clearly outlines the different components and phases of a man's sexual response: erection, arousal, orgasm, and ejaculation. The other three chapters address how to last longer, get fuller and more satisfying erections, and intensify arousal and orgasm.

Since men and women are different physiologically, Sexual Arousal and Women (Part III) contains three chapters of its own. The first chapter in this section describes recent findings about female sexual response, and explores the psychology of arousal. The next two chapters provide methods to deepen arousal and make orgasm much more pleasurable, such as dis-covering personal arousal triggers, and how to have a "gusher."

Finally, the last part of the book explores the many facets of intimacy: bonding, trust, good communication skills, sexual play, healing, and ecstasy. The exercises described in these chapters are to enhance feelings of closeness and connection with your partner, which deepen the joy in your sex life and entire relationship.

You may be a little puzzled that I have placed the chapters on intimacy last. Shouldn't we try to become more intimate before we do sexual exercises? My experience with clients has shown the opposite: learning basic exercises, learning about your own body, and increasing passion and arousal provide the *foundation* for the mutuality and intimacy skills you will develop in the last few chapters.

How to Use This Book

First, read all the way through the book so you understand the nonperformance philosophy behind the exercises and get a feel for them. Then you and your partner can each start on the exercises in Chapter 3, "Learning the Ways of Your Body." You can also do these exercises if you do not have a current sexual partner. Then do the basic partner exercises described in Chapter 4, "Partner Caresses That Kindle Desire."

At this point, you can do whatever progression of exercises you and your partner would like, based on your particular sexual interests. I would suggest going through Chapter 6 on lasting longer for men and then Chapters 10 and 11 on arousal and orgasm for women. After those, you may wish to do the exercises in the chapters on erection and male orgasm, and finally the exercises in the last two chapters on mutuality and intimacy. In my experience, this progression works best because couples often find it easier to do the female arousal exercises if the man has already mastered a high level of ejaculation control.

Alternately, you can identify a goal, such as developing fuller, larger erections. After you do the basic sensate focus exercises in Chapter 3 and understand the arousal process in Chapter 4, you can target the exercises that address your goal in the other chapters.

You can repeat the exercises as many times as you like. Set aside an hour for each session. If you only plan to do each exercise once, you will learn most effectively if you schedule practice sessions one to three times a week. If you do the exercises irregularly, you will forget what you have learned. On the other hand, if you try to do them more than three times a week, you may get burned out.

If you do these exercises one to three times a week, you will certainly see a change in your sexual enjoyment within a month. Most of the changes are gradual, so look for improvement after you do two or three exercises, instead of after each one.

A *Personal* Note

The therapeutic approach I advocate is the culmination of many years of study and clinical work. I have been a professional in the field of sex therapy since 1980, and have a doctoral degree in Health Psychology from the University of California. Health psychologists study the relationship between physical health and mental health, or the mind and body, if you will. Consequently, I take a mind-body approach to human sexuality.

Since receiving my doctorate, I have taught human sexuality at several universities. I have taught techniques similar to the ones described in this book to students who wish to become

marriage and family counselors. I also practice as a sex therapist. I know the techniques described in this book work, because I have taught them to hundreds of clients.

It was out of this experience that I wrote my first book,
*Sexual Healing: A Self-Help Program to Enhance Your Sensuality
and Overcome Common Sexual Problems*. That book was aimed
at people with specific sexual difficulties.

Sexual Pleasure naturally follows. The sensate focus approach and specific techniques in this book can add richness to
anyone's sex life, even ones that are already fulfilling.

I am pleased to share these techniques with you. I *know*
they can work for you and your lover. May the pleasure you
take in each other deepen in the months and years ahead.

Part One
Sensational Sexuality

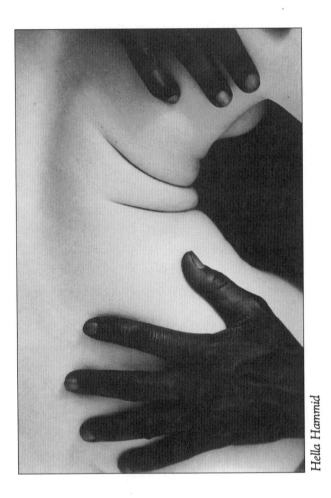

Hella Hammid

Chapter One
The Touch That Transforms Sex

*S*ometimes the simplest ideas have the most power to change our experience. Here is one I would like you to consider: *the feelings in your fingertips and skin are the central elements in satisfying sex.*

If you find this hard to believe, it may be because you have grown used to a way of touching that doesn't give you maximum sensual pleasure.

Sensate focus exercises can change that.

The name may sound somewhat technical, but it is actually self-explanatory. As you do the exercises you *focus* your attention as closely as you can on your *sensations*. This is the essence of the technique. You draw your attention into your body and focus it gently on the places where your skin brushes against your partner's skin, or hair, or fingertips. As the point of your contact shifts, your attention follows. Every time your mind wanders off, you bring it back.

Another essential is that you keep your touch light and very, very *slow*. Being touched in a slow, sensuous way is comforting and relaxing, which is necessary if you are to reach optimal levels of arousal. Bringing your mind and body to a single point of focus adds to that sense of relaxation, and also has the effect of vivifying your experience. This is what gives sensate focus touch the power to transform sex.

The third essential is that you touch for your *own* pleasure. Don't try to turn your partner on. Rather, allow yourself to discover what feels best to you. Paradoxically, this serves your partner, too. When you focus on your own pleasure, there is no pressure on your partner to respond in any specific way, nor on you to "perform." That's why sex therapists call this "nondemand interaction." This type of anxiety-free touch communicates tenderness, caring, and gentleness. It also leaves both of you freer *just to enjoy*.

Sensate focus caresses can be done on any part of the body, including the genitals. They range from the highly sensual to the highly sexual, depending upon which part of the body is being touched. Sensuality is about touch and sensation, not arousal. Sensual touch, however, can *enhance* sexual arousal. I will have you experiment with this kind of touch on yourself first, so that you can explore what pleases you and discover where you are most sensitive. Then you will take turns touching your partner and being touched.

You can touch with your fingertips, your hand, or even with your face, your hair, and the soft undersides of your arms. When you are touching your partner, always maintain skin contact. Lie close to your partner and try not to release a touch, even if you switch hands. If you use lotion or oil for a caress, warm it up in your hand before you apply it, and maintain some contact with your partner if you reapply it.

Now that you understand the basics, let's look more closely at the important ideas behind this sensual touch, and how it is different from the kind of sexual touch you may be used to. You need to be thoroughly familiar with the principles of sensual touch, because you will use them in each of the exercises that follow.

Touch for Your Own Pleasure

The touch used in a sensate focus exercise is called "caressing." In this caress, you touch the skin to get as much *sensation* for yourself as possible. It is not the same type of touch as massage. Massage is a heavy manipulation of body muscles, while caressing gives you and your partner the most acute sense of touching and being touched.

There is no right or wrong way to do a sensate focus exercise. It is almost a "technique-free" technique because everyone has his or her own style of touching. However, certain types of touch are easiest to concentrate on.

Your caress should be light and very, very slow. You can use either long, sweeping strokes or short ones. Try them both and do whatever feels best to you. You and your partner will be able to concentrate best if you touch as slowly as possible. Even if you think you are touching slowly enough, try closing your eyes and cutting your touching speed in half to see if this helps you focus. As you touch, pay attention to temperatures, textures, and shapes on whatever part of the body you are caressing. Remember to touch to make *yourself* feel good and to help your partner focus on your touch.

The best position for any caress is one that allows you to touch with the least amount of physical exertion. If you are going to touch your partner's back, for instance, try lying next to your partner and touching with one hand, rather than straddling your partner.

Focus on Sensations

Recent advances in both psychology and medicine have shown the importance of considering the body and the mind as a whole. Research in sexuality shows that we need to work with the body and mind together to enhance our sexual awareness. Sensate focus exercises reinforce this connection.

During the exercise, both partners concentrate as much as they can on exactly where they are touching or being touched. If you find your mind drifting to something else, catch it and bring it back. If you are touching your partner's face with your fingertips, keep returning your attention to what your fingertips feel. Is the skin smooth or rough? Is your partner tense or relaxed? Do you *like* the feel of the skin?

If you are receiving a sensate focus touch, you also concentrate on the exact point of contact. If your face is being touched, follow the sensations in your skin as your partner's fingertips move across it. Is the touch light enough? What sensations are created from the contact? What other feelings come up, positive or negative? Are you comfortable with them? If not, can you relax and let yourself be comfortable with them?

By noticing these sensations, you increase your awareness of the amount of sensation you can feel—and therefore, the amount of pleasure available to you.

Realize that distractions always occur during a sensate focus exercise. You might hear a noise in the house or find yourself wondering what to make for dinner, or what you really should have said during negotiations at work. During any given exercise, it doesn't matter if your mind drifts off fifty times—the important thing is that you recognize that you are thinking about something else and consciously bring your mind back to the touch. Don't criticize yourself for not being able to maintain your focus. Everybody gets distracted. You will become better at staying focused each time you practice these exercises.

It is a little easier to concentrate during a sensate focus exercise than during usual sex, because most of the exercises are nonverbal. This leaves both of you free to concentrate 100 percent on the touch without distractions.

Stay in the Here and Now

Each time you bring your mind back to the sensation, you bring it back to the present moment. When you are *touching*, this means that you are focusing on the body area you are touching right now, not the area you will be touching a few minutes from now or the area you just touched. If you are *receiving* a sensate focus exercise, staying in the here and now means focusing on the body area your partner is touching now, not the area that he or she touched five minutes ago or the area that you wish he or she would touch. If you have thoughts such as, "I wish she'd go back to my chin," or even, "When are we going to have sex?" then you are failing to concentrate fully. When you realize this, consciously bring your attention back to the point of contact between your skin and your partner's fingertips.

Staying in the here and now also means that you are focusing on the sensual or sexual encounter you are having right now, rather than one you may have had in the past or that you may have in the future. Sex, like life, happens in the here and now. Dwelling on thoughts of sexual encounters in the past will distract you. Speculating about what will happen in the future may make you anxious and unable to enjoy a caress. Keeping in the here and now is the key to pleasure: it brings you back into your body so your mind can register *all* the exquisite sensations of being touched in a loving way.

Eliminate Expectations from Your Touch

When you do sensate focus exercises, there is no pressure to perform in a particular way. This nondemand style of interaction is the result of several conscious choices, which help you to fully experience pleasure. One is to take the pressure off yourself. Another is to take the pressure off your partner. The third, which I will discuss first, is to allow yourself to experience the exercises as both an active participant and passive participant.

Active and Passive Roles

Most sensate focus exercises for couples start with one person as the passive partner and one as the active partner, and then the partners switch roles. This helps eliminate performance pressure and minimizes the distractions so you can concentrate on touching or being touched.

When you are the active partner, do the caress as instructed and try to keep your attention on exactly where your fingertips or skin touches your partner's skin. Touch for your own pleasure. Don't worry about what your partner may be thinking or feeling and do not speak to your partner during the exercise or ask for feedback. Assume that the caress feels good. If something bothers your partner, he or she will tell you. Your only task when you are active is to focus on your own sensations. When you are done, tell your partner.

When you are the passive partner, lie in a comfortable position. Relax any muscles that feel tense. Focus on the sensations you receive when your partner touches you. Mentally follow his or her hand as it caresses your body. Let your partner know if he or she is doing something that hurts or bothers you. If not, do not say anything or give any feedback. Just allow yourself to soak up the sensations like a sponge. You don't have any responsibility except to focus on what you are feeling.

You may initially have some resistance to remaining completely passive. *I urge you to try.* You may find that being in this unfamiliar role and allowing yourself just to receive is quite enjoyable.

Not having constant verbal feedback from your partner may seem frustrating or unnatural at first, but it will help you learn which sensations and touches you like. Dividing activities into two specific roles also helps you learn more about your own body—and your partner's—than if you were instructed to touch each other at the same time. By concentrating totally on where your skin touches your partner's skin, you will become fully involved and present in what is happening. Although only one partner is active at a time, your point of focus is the same. You will find this more sensually arousing than when you and your partner do different activities at the same time. This passive role/active role approach also fosters an attitude of sharing and trust.

When sex therapists first started having their clients do sensate focus exercises, the instructions were somewhat different than the ones you just read. Sex therapists used to tell their clients, "When you are active, try to please your partner. When you are passive, tell your partner everything you like and don't like." They found soon enough, however, that this could create a lot of performance pressure.

From working with clients, my colleagues and I have found that when people are instructed to touch for their own pleasure, they enjoy more and learn more—and so does their partner. If you start your touching practice with exercises that use the active and passive roles, you will actually become more confident about touching your partner than if you engaged in touching mutually.

Taking Pressure off Your Partner

When you are active during a sensate focus caress, don't worry about how your partner will respond. If he or she becomes aroused during the caress, that's fine, but there should be no *expectation* that your partner will become aroused, stay aroused, have an erection, have an orgasm, have an ejaculation, or hold anything back. This is why we call these sensate focus exercises "nondemand" interactions.

It is normal and loving to want to know that your partner

is enjoying himself or herself. However, the problem with expecting your partner to respond in a certain way is that your expectations are communicated nonverbally even if you do not say anything. You don't have to say, "Are you aroused?" or "Did you come?" for your partner to feel pressure. When you have expectations, your touch changes subtly and your partner can pick this up. You and your partner will then both have a difficult time focusing on your feelings—focusing on the touch.

Taking Pressure off Yourself

We often put even more pressure on ourselves than we do on our partners. During a sensate focus exercise, try not to have any expectations about how you will feel or respond. There is no requirement that you respond in any particular way during an exercise. Although some of the sensate focus exercises teach you how to recognize different levels of arousal or erection, *there is never any demand that you have a particular level of arousal or erection during any exercise.* It is important to remember this when you come to these exercises; knowing and being aware of different levels for *yourself* does not mean having to reach particular levels for the exercises to be successful.

Some people become concerned because they do not experience sexual arousal during some of the sensate focus exercises. Don't be. Many of the exercises are sensual, not sexual— they are about touch and sensation, not arousal. For example, I have had clients who did not experience a genital caress as particularly sexual, and I have also had clients who experienced a face caress as sexual.

If you feel arousal during an exercise, don't interfere with it, just let it happen. Do not try to increase your arousal, do not try to fight it off, and do not try to control it. Just take a deep breath and enjoy it, even if it goes all the way to orgasm.

Benefits of Touching

Why learn to touch in this way? Research has shown that touching and being touched provide a number of benefits beyond the obvious increase in sexual enjoyment.

The first benefit is relaxation. Certain types of touch help our bodies relax, whether we are active or passive. Touching and relaxation go together. In fact, touching can actually bring physical healing. The "laying on of hands" has been used in many cultures throughout the world to cure physical illnesses.

Much of the research on touch and health has been brought together by Ashley Montagu in his classic book, *Touching*. Montagu describes the effect of skin contact on the mental and physical health of people of all ages. His book shows that touch is vitally important for humans, as well as for other animals. Infant monkeys, for example, deprived of touch have sexual problems later in life. Human infants deprived of contact have higher death rates than those who are touched. In human adults, being touched has been shown to lower heart rate and blood pressure, and to reduce the effects of stress. Touching may also have a positive effect on our immune system.

Although touch obviously has benefits for adults, there is no research that shows that adults *need* touch. But there is no reason to think that our need to be touched ends with infancy or childhood. The desire to be held or touched is a strong motivation for engaging in sexual activities. For many of us, and especially for men, sexual encounters are the only situations in which we are allowed to touch other human beings or enjoy being touched by them.

Touching also makes it easier to share feelings. Patients who are touched in the genital area by doctors or nurses during a physical examination often spontaneously confide personal sexual information. It seems that being touched in intimate areas brings intimate thoughts and feelings to the surface.

Being touched has been shown to have a positive effect on adults in medical settings as well. For example, in one study, patients who were touched by nurses recovered faster than those who were not touched. It is not known *how* touching helps people get better. It could be that touching promotes relaxation and indirectly affects the immune system. Or, it could be that the act of touching communicates the expectation that the patient will get well.

Some of us grew up in families that touched and others did not. Whether you are naturally comfortable with touching and being touched or not, the exercises in this book—which start out nonsexual and gradually proceed to the more sexual—will help you get the wonderful touching you need for relaxation, comfort, and physical and mental well-being. They will develop your confidence in, desire for, and appreciation and enjoyment of touch.

In the next chapter, we will look at how relaxation makes us even more responsive to the pleasure of the sensual touch.

Chapter Two

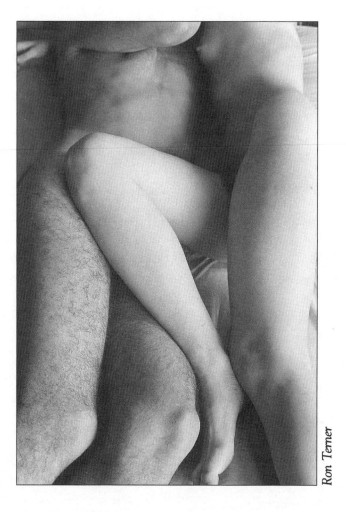

Ron Terner

*Relaxation to Heighten
Your Pleasure Response*

F eeling tired and tense hardly creates the right setting for great sex. Yet, that's how most of us feel
after a typical week of meeting deadlines at work,
running the kids around town, and keeping the clutter from
overtaking the house. Since most of us are usually so keyed-up,
it's a miracle we feel much of anything when we reach for an
intimate moment with our partners.

Optimal pleasure requires us to be deeply relaxed. That
is why it is so important to take time to relax before making
love. Sex therapists know that relaxation is crucial to sexual
arousal and that anxiety, the opposite of relaxation, can stop
arousal cold.

If it has been a long time since you've felt *really* relaxed,
you might need to be reminded about what it feels like. During
deep relaxation, you breathe deeply. Your muscles relax and
your heart slows to a gentler pace. You may find you have few
thoughts at all, or that they just drift by randomly, without
taking hold. This is the body's relaxation response. Your body
uses this "rest break" to conserve energy for a later time.

The benefits of making time to relax this deeply are well
known. Relaxation training is considered a good preventive
strategy against physical and mental illness. It has also been

shown to improve conditions as varied as cancer and heart disease, and to alleviate mental disorders caused by anxiety, stress, and mood dysfunctions. Fortunately, sensate focus exercises provide the same relaxation benefits as many other kinds of relaxation practices.

The Physiology of Relaxation

To learn how to activate the relaxation response, you need to know a little bit about the autonomic nervous system, which is responsible for speeding up or slowing down your physical responses. The autonomic nervous system regulates those body functions such as heartbeat and digestion, which were once considered beyond our voluntary control. However, in the last few decades, we have learned that it is possible to consciously influence these processes. Much of this knowledge has come from studying practitioners of yoga and other meditative disciplines, who have trained in mastering these body functions.

The autonomic nervous system has two separate and contradictory branches. One of these is the sympathetic nervous system. If you are faced with some immediate danger, this system springs into action and helps your body mobilize the energy to either fight or run away. When this happens, your eyes dilate, your heart rate speeds up, and your breathing and blood pressure increase dramatically. Another important effect is that blood flows immediately to your limbs. This response developed evolutionally because those parts of your body needed the extra resources to face the "danger" creating your anxiety. The sympathetic nervous system is activated very rapidly. It only takes seconds for the blood to flow away from the center of your body and out to your arms and legs.

When you think about the direction of the blood flow during this "fight or flight" response, it probably becomes clear how anxiety can interfere with your sexual response. When you are anxious, blood flows *away* from the center of your body, including the genitals. When you are relaxed, blood flows toward the center of the body.

This quick-response system is useful if you really are in some kind of danger. But in these stressful times, most of us have sympathetic nervous systems that are a little too active. Some of us experience that sympathetic nervous system surge when we have to take a test, speak in public, or even have sex!

The parasympathetic nervous system is the other branch of the autonomic nervous system. It is responsible for slowing your body down so you can conserve energy. This system is active when your body is taking care of its life-sustaining processes, like digestion. When the parasympathetic nervous system is "on" you feel deeply relaxed. This is also the system that is active when you feel deeply aroused.

Although the sympathetic or anxiety response happens almost instantaneously, the relaxation response is rather slow. These two systems are not able to operate simultaneously. As we know, we cannot feel *anxious* and *relaxed* at the same time. However, as you will see later, these two systems can actually work *together*; they can complement each other.

Because of how the two nervous systems function, it is impossible to turn off the sympathetic nervous system by trying to turn it off. If you try to turn it off, you will become more, rather than less, anxious. The only way to turn off the anxiety is to turn on the parasympathetic or relaxation system. Sensate focus exercises provide you with one way of doing this.

Increasing Your Relaxation Response

With practice, you can consciously activate your relaxation response within about five minutes. One great way to do this is to close your eyes, lie quietly without moving, and take several slow, deep breaths. Realize that it may take several minutes of this for your whole body to relax. Your nervous system tends to take longer to slow down than it does to speed up.

This relaxed state has been described very well by Dr. Herbert Benson in his book, *The Relaxation Response*. According to Dr. Benson, there are four things necessary to reach this relaxed state:

1. A quiet environment

2. A mental device (like a favorite prayer or phrase, or a number you keep focusing on, again and again)

3. A comfortable physical position

4. A receptive or passive attitude

I would like to add a fifth item to Dr. Benson's list: *a predictable activity*.

The sensate focus exercises satisfy each of these conditions. You always do them in a quiet room. Focusing on your sensations and the exact point of contact gives you the "mental device" to keep your mind occupied, so it is less likely to get caught up in anxious thoughts. As you do these exercises, you and your partner will make yourselves physically comfortable. You will each take turns being the passive partner, in which your only concern is to focus on sensations. Finally, if you do each exercise as described, you will know exactly what is going to happen and this will further relax you.

The Brain, Relaxation, and Arousal

Your mind functions differently when you are relaxed than when you are anxious. Your brain constantly produces mild electrical activity, usually called brain waves. When you are in a state of alert wakefulness, your brain produces fast waves called beta waves. Waves characteristic of a more relaxed state are slower waves called alpha waves. The best way to induce alpha waves is to lie down, relax all of your muscles, slow your breathing down, close your eyes, and let your mind drift without focusing on anything in particular.

During some of the exercises described in this book, you may find that you relax so much that you actually reach a very advanced relaxation state or alpha state. In this state, you may feel as if you are floating or drifting. It is a wonderful feeling, but you do not *need* to be in this deeply relaxed state to do the exercises.

When you begin an exercise, you may relax into the alpha state. At this phase the parasympathetic nervous system is activated. Then, if the exercise includes genital contact, you will start to become aroused. As you reach higher and higher levels of arousal, the sympathetic nervous system starts to come into play. At the point of orgasm, it is the sympathetic nervous system that is activated. The body changes at that point include heavy breathing, muscle tension, and increased heart rate and blood pressure. At orgasm, all of this tension comes to a peak and is discharged, resulting in an intense feeling of release.

Sexual activity is one of the very few experiences a human can have in which the sympathetic nervous system and the parasympathetic nervous system work together. Sexual arousal and orgasm depend on a delicate interplay and balance between these two systems. But none of it will work unless you start out in a relaxed state. That is why so many of the exercises in this book stress the importance of relaxation.

There is another change that takes place in your body when you reach extremely high levels of sexual arousal and *stay* there for a while. The combination of controlled physical activity, heavy breathing, and sexual arousal generally produces the release of endorphins. You may have heard of endorphins: the pleasure chemicals produced by the brain. Heroin and other similar drugs work because we already have these receptor sites for pleasure chemicals in our brains. When you release endorphins due to sexual arousal, you may experience an altered or transcendent state of consciousness. These endorphins can dull or even eliminate pain, so sexual arousal is a natural painkiller.

Relaxation and Touching

Certain types of touch activate the parasympathetic nervous system and certain types of touch activate the sympathetic nervous system. The type of touching you learn to do in the sensate focus exercises described in this book activates the parasympathetic nervous system—your relaxation response.

Sensate focus touching is slow, very light, and soothing. It starts on the arms and legs and moves to the genitals. Touching or being touched with this caressing style will activate the relaxation response for both you and your partner.

On the other hand, being touched in a threatening, unpredictable, mechanical, or heavy way makes us anxious. Being touched in an intimate body area also makes us anxious if it is sudden or inappropriate. So, when you do the exercises in this book, take care to touch your partner in a way that will trigger relaxation and not anxiety. If you are passive during an exercise and your partner's touch is so heavy that it triggers anxiety, tell your partner.

Anxious Thoughts

Your thoughts also contribute to your feelings of relaxation or anxiety. Your thoughts can activate either the sympathetic nervous system or the parasympathetic nervous system. Fearful or worried thoughts are the mental component of anxiety, whereas slow thoughts contribute to relaxation.

There are several thought patterns that can contribute to anxiety during sex and can short-circuit your relaxation response. The most common of these thought patterns are spectatoring, racing thoughts, and performance thoughts.

Spectatoring is a term coined by Masters and Johnson. It refers to a habit of mentally watching yourself and evaluating or grading your performance during sexual activity. A person who is spectatoring is constantly monitoring and making mental notes about sexual arousal instead of *experiencing* sexual arousal. For example, a man might find himself thinking, "She's touching my penis. It's starting to feel a little hard. What if she—oh, no, I'm losing my erection." Spectatoring often takes on an obsessive quality; that is, a person feels *compelled* to consciously monitor what is going on.

As you do the sensate focus exercises, you will learn to focus on what is happening sexually and sensually instead of worrying about it. You'll become more accustomed to *experiencing* what is happening instead of *thinking* about it. Gradually, spectatoring will cease to occur.

If you have **racing thoughts**, it means your mind is working very fast and jumping from thought to thought, and not staying on any one topic or idea. Many people have this tendency, but I see it most in highly intelligent people, who have cultivated the ability to switch quickly from topic to topic. Although this is advantageous in the work arena, it can get in the way of enjoying sex.

Fortunately, this is one of the easiest types of anxiety-related thoughts to deal with. As you start to do some of the exercises described in this book, and you begin to caress, the pace at which you do the caress will actually slow your thoughts down. And when you are the passive partner in an exercise and are most susceptible to racing thoughts, your partner's slow touch will set the speed for your thoughts.

Thinking of sex as work or as a performance can also interfere with your sexual enjoyment. Have you ever caught yourself thinking, "Darn, I was unable to perform," or, "Great—I achieved an orgasm"? Thinking of sex in this way keeps you in your head rather than in your body. You become so focused on the goal of "orgasm," that you hardly pay attention to the sensuous feelings throughout your body.

Probably the most damaging type of anxious thoughts are the performance fears that lead to what sex therapists call "performance anxiety." These are thoughts that cause you to worry that someone is watching you or that something other than pleasure depends on the outcome of a sexual encounter. I have worked with people whose whole sense of self-esteem was riding on their sexual performance. If the encounter was not perfect, they were devastated. Others depended on sexual performance to build an image as a good lover, or to keep a marriage together. You can imagine how much tension this can add to sex.

Performance thoughts also occur when you start to wonder if your partner is enjoying himself or herself or what he or she is thinking. Other typical performance thoughts include, "Is he watching me?" "Am I doing a good job?" "Why don't I have an erection yet?" "Why hasn't she come?" or "Was his previous lover better than I am?"

These kinds of thoughts have the power to shut down your sexual response immediately. Many sex therapists believe that performance anxiety is either directly or indirectly responsible for the majority of sexual problems.

If sex has been a work or performance activity for you all your life, do not expect to change these feelings overnight. It will take some practice for you to view sex as a pleasure activity rather than a situation in which you have to achieve. But try to remember that sex is for your enjoyment. The rules that apply in achievement situations—"If I try hard, I will succeed," or "If I move faster, I will succeed"—do not apply here. In fact, they're usually counterproductive.

To enjoy the exercises this book, you need to go as slowly as you can. You need to stop "trying." *Working* at an exercise instead of *experiencing* it won't allow you to enjoy the exercise.

If you do the exercises regularly, you will find that they actually help you decrease your performance-oriented thoughts. They do this by teaching you how to focus on your own enjoyment before you have any activity with a partner. They do this by having you focus on your sensations, which occupies your mind. They do this by showing you how to interact with your partner's response so that you have no questions or doubts.

But What If the Pressure Is Real?

Not all thoughts that cause anxiety and performance pressure are "in your head." What if the reason you are feeling performance pressure is because the pressure is really there? What if your partner is the one putting pressure on you, rather than you putting it on yourself?

People can pressure each other in both subtle and not-so-subtle ways, not all of which are verbal. Verbal pressure is usually fairly easy to recognize. It can take the form of questions such as, "Why don't you have an erection yet?" or "Aren't you going to come pretty soon?" or even, "Did you come?"

Nonverbal pressure is more subtle. Your sexual partner cannot read your mind. However, he or she can definitely tell if you are thinking about something else or wishing you were somewhere else. A facial expression or even a sigh can convey that you are bored with an activity or that you are somehow disappointed in your own response or your partner's response.

How can you deal with this? If the problem during a sexual encounter has been that you feel pressured to perform and are giving and receiving nonverbal cues, try the exercises in this book. Learning to pay attention to your own sensations, not worrying about your partner, and improving your communication when you talk about sex will alleviate these performance issues. If you are under constant verbal pressure from your partner, however, you both should consider professional counseling.

With the principles of sensate focus and relaxation in mind, you are ready to actually begin some caressing—to learn the ways of your body and the power of your arousal.

Chapter Three

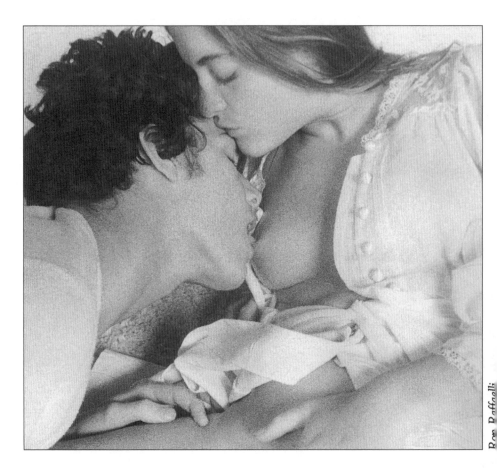

Ron Raffaelli

Learning the Ways of Your Body

Now that you are familiar with the basic principles of sensate focus, you are ready for some exercises that will teach you more about your body and its natural sexual responses. Practice these sensual and sexual exercises yourself before you go on to the partner exercises. I would like you to practice the exercises for breathing and control of the puboccocygeus (PC) and pelvic muscles every day from now on, and to practice the self-caressing, "peaking," and "plateauing" exercises at least once, but more if you can. Taking time alone to explore your own response to touch so you can learn how to bring yourself to deeper and deeper levels of arousal will add immeasurably to the excitement you create with your partner.

This is particularly true for women. In my practice, I see many women who have never really touched their genitals or even looked at them. Few women explore their bodies enough to discover what really turns them on. Often this lack of self-knowledge is the only thing stopping them from becoming aroused enough to reach orgasm. Fortunately, this is easy to remedy. For such women, the "peaking" exercises can radically change their experience of intercourse. These exercises build sexual "charge" and make orgasm that much more explosive.

I want to stress, however, that each of these exercises is beneficial for both men and women. The ideas of pleasing *yourself*, knowing your *own* body, and learning about *your* own natural sexual responses are so important that I have emphasized them throughout the book. Learn to trust yourself and your own feelings.

The first few exercises below condition your body for pleasure and the later exercises help you discover your natural arousal patterns. These are the first steps on the path to heightened sexual pleasure.

Exercise 1
Belly Breathing

Here's a simple breathing exercise to do for ten minutes each day. I start with this one because proper breathing is essential for sexual arousal. In fact, it is impossible to become sexually aroused if you are holding your breath. If you do this type of breathing exercise every day, it will lower your heart rate and blood pressure, and it will allow you to relax so that you can do the rest of the exercises that follow.

This exercise is called "belly breathing." To start, lie comfortably on your back. Place one hand on your abdomen. Slowly breathe in through your mouth and then slowly exhale. Your stomach should rise and fall with this breath.

Do two or three belly breaths and then breathe normally for a couple of minutes. Then belly breathe again. While belly breathing, pause for three seconds between breathing out and breathing in. Don't pause between breathing in and breathing out—the inhale and exhale should be one continuous process.

Exercise 2
Relaxation Breathing

If you are especially anxious or have a lot of stress in your life, also try the following breathing exercise. Blow all the air out of your lungs through your nose rather rapidly. Now take all the air you can back in through your nose, *slowly*. Think of it as caressing the inside of your lungs with air. Relax your stomach muscles. As soon as the air is all in your lungs, start breathing it back out slowly. Don't hold your breath at all.

Your breath is now under your conscious control. Do this five or six times. It will slow down your heart rate and lower your blood pressure. This simple breathing exercise, if done right, can give you all the relaxation you need to do the exercises in this book.

Exercise 3
The Daily PC Muscle Exercise

The other daily exercise that I would like you to do involves a particular group of muscles in your pelvic area. The full name for it is the pubococcygeus or pubococcygeal muscle group, but it is often called the PC muscle for short. This muscle group runs from the pubic bone in front to the tailbone in the rear and supports the pelvic floor.

In men, this is the muscle that spasms when ejaculation occurs. In women, this is the muscle that spasms during orgasm and gives the vagina a feeling of tightness.

A strong PC muscle contributes to your pleasure in sex in several ways. If you exercise it daily, you will build the muscle mass in the pelvic area, which will increase the amount of blood flowing to your genitals and allow for more pleasurable sensations during arousal. In addition, a strong PC muscle can tighten the vagina and makes orgasm and ejaculation more enjoyable. An added benefit is that a strong PC muscle often prevents bladder and prostate problems. In fact, correcting bladder problems in pregnant women was how this muscle was first "discovered." In the chapters ahead, I'll give you more specifics on working with the PC muscle to heighten your arousal.

To exercise the muscle, you must first learn to identify it. Here's how:

Men, to locate your PC muscle, lightly place one or two fingers behind your testicles. Pretend that you are urinating and want to stop the flow by tightening an internal muscle. That is the PC muscle. You may notice that your penis and testicles move a little as you tighten the muscle.

Women, to locate your PC muscle, either place one or two fingers lightly on the inner vaginal lips or insert a finger about one inch into the vagina. Now squeeze as if you were urinating and wanted to stop the flow. The muscle that tightens as you do this is the PC muscle. Try to flex only that small muscle and keep your thigh and abdomen muscles relaxed.

Now that you know where the PC muscle is, here is the daily PC muscle exercise I want you to do. Three times a day, flex the PC muscle and hold it for about two seconds. Then release. Don't hold your breath while you are holding the muscle in. Just breathe normally. Start with six exercises, then gradually build up to twenty-five repetitions over four months. The great thing about this exercise is that you can practice any time of the day. You can do the exercises during your morning shower, immediately after you use the toilet, while you are watching television, or during any activity that you repeat every day.

There are two common mistakes that people make when beginning these exercises. The first is to overdo the repetitions by doing too many at one time or too frequently during the day.

Like any other muscle, the PC can become sore. The second mistake is to squeeze other muscles instead of the PC. When you do PC muscle exercises, your stomach, buttocks, thigh, and abdominal muscles should not tense at all. Of course, they probably will at first, but work on relaxing them so you can isolate the PC muscle.

You do not need to keep your finger on the PC muscle when you exercise it. You will be able to feel it move internally. If you have trouble isolating the PC muscle from other pelvic muscles, either keep your finger on it the first few times you do the exercises, or exercise the muscle while you urinate and see if you can stop the flow.

It takes about three weeks of daily exercises for your PC muscle to get in shape. Once it is in shape, you should still exercise it every day to keep it strong and enjoy the benefits.

Exercise 4
The Advanced PC Muscle Exercise

After you have been doing 25 simple PC muscle exercises for three weeks, try the following more difficult exercise: add 10 slow repetitions. Try to tense the muscle for a count of five seconds, hold for five seconds, and then release or push out on the muscle for five seconds. Again, it may take several days or weeks to work up to 10 repetitions. That's okay. Just do as many as you can.

Because of how much they contribute to pelvic health and sexual pleasure, I cannot overemphasize the importance of PC exercises. When you begin to experience the results, you will get hooked on them, too.

Exercise 5
Pelvic Thrusts and Rolls

The next two exercises can help you loosen up the muscles in your pelvic area, especially your hips, thighs, and buttocks. They are also good for your back. A flexible pelvis can help you do more sexual positions and allow you to become more sexually aroused. Too much muscle tension in the pelvic area limits your arousal and can interfere with sensations of sexual pleasure.

Pelvic thrusts can be done either lying down or standing. To do them standing, plant your feet about shoulder width apart and gently but firmly rock or tilt your pelvis from back to front without moving any other parts of your body.

If you are lying down, put your knees up and rock or tilt your buttocks slowly up and down so they are the only part of you that moves off the floor. Do this at a comfortable pace and repeat about 20 times. Keep your other muscles relaxed and breathe evenly.

If you want to practice these pelvic thrusts while walking, thrust your pelvis forward with each step.

Pelvic rolls are similar to thrusts. Either lying or standing, move your hips in a continuous rolling motion. If you have difficulty getting the hang of this, you might want to try using a hula hoop. Practice rolls at different speeds, and practice some as slowly as you can. Combine thrusts and rolls and try to do them for five or ten minutes a day. Do them to music if it feels good. Try closing your eyes so you can really feel your body.

Enhancing Touch with
Sensuous Oils and Lubricants

In the following exercise and in most of the exercises throughout this book, I will suggest you use an oil, lotion, or lubricant
for your caress. Oils and lubricants will increase your pleasure
reception—the sense of a touch seems to linger longer and
more acutely. They also enhance the sensations you feel by
keeping your skin moist and preventing your touch from grab-
bing or sticking to the skin. For many of the advanced exercises
during which you enjoy prolonged stroking, you will need this
additional lubrication to maintain pleasurable friction.

I prefer to use mineral oil because it stays warm on the
body and tends to last longer. Water-based lubricants, such as
K-Y Jelly, are safe to use with condoms, but they tend to feel
cooler and do not last as long. Recently, lubricants have come
on the market that simulate vaginal lubrication. These can be
very enjoyable, but also do not tend to last long on the body.

Some couples enjoy using scented or edible oils and lotions because they spark other senses and can be sexy and fun.
Different scents have been known to have relaxing or enervat-
ing effects, which the practice of aromatherapy is based on.
These types of oils are usually available in adult boutiques or
specialty bath shops. Other couples prefer to use an entirely
natural lubricant, such as vegetable oil, which has no scent and
is very compatible with the body.

There are many good lubricants available to you. The lotions and oils you choose can affect and enhance the sensations
you and your lover feel, so experiment with them to find the
ones you enjoy most and that work best for you. If you do try a
new one, start out with a small amount, because it may cause
irritation. If it does, stop using it and try something else later.
You can also try varying your oils and lotions according to the

exercises and your mood, to see what sensual pleasures they bring out. Diversity, after all, is the spice of life!

Exercise 6
The Simple Self-Caress

Now you will learn to practice the basic sensate focus techniques you read about in Chapter 1. Before you do any touching exercises with your partner, you'll practice first on your own body. This is a very important part of the sensate focus program. Again, I strongly recommend that you practice self-caress techniques and get to know your own sensual responses before you move on to practicing with a partner.

Before you begin, have some baby oil or other lotion handy. Choose a small area of your body, such as your arm, chest, or thigh for your first caress. Put some lotion on your hand and slowly touch yourself. Focus on the exact point of contact between your hand and your body. If your mind starts to wander off to something else, bring it back to exactly how your skin feels.

Touch yourself slowly and lightly on the skin surface— don't massage the muscles. Remember to breathe evenly as you do the caress. Pay attention to the temperature and texture of your skin. Is it warm or cold, smooth or rough, firm or soft? If you have trouble focusing, slow down. Spend at least ten to fifteen minutes on this caress. If you have difficulty or become agitated, anxious, or uncomfortable during the simple self-caress, *don't* go any further. If your anxiety is particularly bad, you may want to see a therapist, discuss what may be happening, and follow his or her advice about what to do next.

Exercise 7
The Genital Self-Caress

After you have practiced the simple self-caress a few times and feel comfortable with it, you are now ready to do a similar caress on your genitals. *This is not the same as masturbation.* You will just caress your genitals slowly so that you can learn what kind of touch you prefer on your genitals. Allow about fifteen minutes for this exercise.

Before you do any exercise where you are touching your genitals or your partner's, and especially when you are inserting a finger into the vagina, be sure to clean your hands, trim your nails, and make sure the area under your nails is clean. For this particular exercise, you will also need some baby oil or another lubricant.

Women, to do this, lie down or sit naked in a comfortable position. Put some baby oil on your fingers and slowly begin to touch your inner thighs and your vaginal lips. Remember to breathe and keep your pelvic muscles, including the PC muscle, relaxed. Slowly stroke your clitoris and inner lips, and then insert a finger into your vagina.

Focus on the point of contact between your hand and your genitals. If your mind starts to wander off to something else, bring it back to the exact point of contact.

Pay attention to the temperature, texture, and shape of your vaginal lips and the area inside. If you become aroused during this caress or have an orgasm, that is fine, but it is not the goal. Don't try to make it happen, don't force it, and don't push it away. Just experience it. Whatever happens is all part of getting in touch with your *pleasure*—enjoying yourself and learning about your own body.

Men, to do this, sit or lie naked in a comfortable position. Use some baby oil or lotion on your fingers. Slowly begin to stroke the skin of your penis and scrotum. Remember to go very slowly; this is not a masturbation stroke. Don't try to get an erection but if you have one, that's okay.

Concentrate on the exact point of contact between your hand and your genitals. Pay attention to the temperature, texture, and shape of your penis and scrotum. If your mind wanders off to something else, slow your touch down and bring your mind back to the point of contact. Remember to breathe and keep your pelvic muscles, including the PC muscle, relaxed.

If you wish to have an orgasm and ejaculation after you have spent fifteen minutes doing this caress, go ahead. Don't force yourself to have one, but don't fight it off if it happens.

Practice each of these self-caressing exercises at least once, but preferably a few times. Repeat them as often as you like. Caressing yourself in this way will teach you to focus on touch, to breathe deeply, and to relax your muscles—the three most important aspects of arousal.

Exercise 8
"Solo" Peaking

Peaking is a process in which you caress your own genitals and learn to modulate your arousal so that it goes up and down in a series of peaks and valleys that are under your control. This increases your staying power and builds up sexual charge.

The first step to peaking is arousal awareness.

Before you learn to peak, you have to be able to recognize how sexually aroused you are. One convenient way to do this is to think of your sexual arousal on a scale from 1 to 10. I know this may seem too clinical and that it may appear to contradict what I said earlier about getting away from a performance orientation. Please don't get the impression that I am asking you to evaluate yourself in any way. Rather, these numbers are to help you *describe* your sexual response. The idea is not to see how high you can go, but to help you become aware of the difference in how you feel at each level. In other words, reaching a "9" is not better than reaching a "3," or vice versa.

I use a number scale because most of us are familiar with the phrase, "on a scale of 1 to 10." Alternately, you might think of a musical scale, in which the notes get higher and higher. We'll be using this arousal scale throughout the book, and I promise it will get easier to work with. After you get used to it, the numbers will just drop away and you'll be left with the sensations. Men, remember, this scale describes how aroused you *feel*, not how strong your erection is.

On this 1 to 10 scale, a 1 is no arousal and a 10 is orgasm. Consider a twinge feeling in the genital area a 2 or 3. A 4 is a steady low level of arousal. A 5 or 6 is a medium level of arousal. By the time you reach level 7 or 8, you may be feeling a little short of breath, or you may feel your heart pound or your face flush. A 9 is the point right before orgasm, and a 10 is the release of orgasm.

Peaking Exercise #1   The point of this exercise is to help you become aware of your arousal level.

Begin a slow genital self-caress as you did in the previous exercise. Caress yourself exactly as you did last time, paying attention to the point of contact, breathing, and relaxing.

Every five minutes or so, ask yourself, "What level do I feel I am at now?" Don't try to reach any particular level of arousal, just notice it and try to estimate your arousal level on that 1 to 10 scale. Don't try to manipulate your arousal level in any way.

Caress your genitals in a way that you like and remember to go slowly to make it easier to stay focused. If you want to have an orgasm at the end of this first exercise, go ahead.

Peaking Exercise #2   In this second exercise you will actually "peak."

To begin, caress your genitals until you think you are just past the twinging stage. Then stop the stimulation and allow yourself to go back to level 1. Now start caressing again and this time go up to level 5, or about halfway to orgasm.

Stop the stimulation and allow your arousal level to go down a couple of levels. Repeat this cycle a few times and try peaking at levels 6, 7, 8, 9. Spend about five minutes per peak, including both the up and down phases. Do the exercise for about twenty minutes. You can conclude it with an orgasm if you wish, but it is not necessary.

Try not to forget the basics. Pay attention to the exact place where your hands are caressing your genitals. Be lovingly slow with your touch. Breathe and keep your muscles, including the PC muscle, relaxed.

Repeat this exercise at least once a week until you feel comfortable spending twenty minutes at it and peaking up to level 8.

In this and the following exercises, allow plenty of time for your arousal to go down, even though you may be tempted to go all the way to orgasm and skip the exercise.

You may find that the peaking practice makes your orgasm stronger, if you decide to have one. The whole process seems to allow for the optimal release of the endorphins we talked about in Chapter 2. This gradual buildup of sexual energy that happens during the peaking process will help your body prepare for the exercises you will do with your partner later in the book.

Exercise 9
"Solo" Plateauing

Plateauing is an advanced form of peaking in which you allow your arousal to go up to a certain level and stay there for a period of time, from a few seconds to as long as a couple of minutes. You do this by using several techniques you have already learned, and a couple of new ones. The techniques are breathing, pelvic movements, switching focus, and using the PC muscle. I recommend you practice using them one at a time, so that you can get each technique down pat before you add the next one.

While this may seem complicated at first because of all the numbers involved, remember that you already have experience recognizing your arousal levels from the peaking exercises.

Plateauing Exercise #1   Begin with a genital caress. Remember to caress in a slow, sensate focus style. Breathe and keep your pelvic muscles relaxed.

Comfortably allow your arousal to go up halfway to orgasm. Try to plateau at this level, which is level 5, using changes in your breathing. As you reach a point a little above level 5, slowly take two deep belly breaths. This will allow your arousal to go down.

When your arousal level goes down a bit to 4, speed up your breathing almost to panting. This will cause your arousal level to go back up. See if you can hover between 4 and 5 for thirty seconds or more just by changing your breathing. The technique here is to slow your breathing down to lower your arousal and speed it up if you want your arousal to go up.

Plateauing Exercise #2   In this exercise, you practice using changes in your pelvic movements to help you plateau. Try to plateau at level 6 this time.

To begin, caress your genitals again and allow your arousal to increase. Start slow pelvic rolls and thrusts, alternating the two movements, when you reach level 3 or 4. This will increase your arousal.

When you reach a point beyond level 6, slow or stop your pelvic movements until you go back down below level 6. When you are a little below 6, speed up your pelvic movements until you go up beyond level 6. See if you can plateau at level 6 for thirty seconds or more, just using changes in your pelvic movements. The basic technique is to speed up or put more energy into your pelvic movements to become more aroused, and slow down your pelvic movements to become less aroused. Repeat this exercise until you it becomes second nature to modulate your arousal by moving your pelvis.

Plateauing Exercise #3   This exercise uses changes in your focus in order to plateau. During any kind of sexual activity, it is possible to focus on a number of different things that are going on. In the previous exercise, I had you focus on the exact point of contact where you are touching yourself. Now we will work on touching one area and focusing on another area.

Caress your genitals until you reach level 6 again. Slowly continue to caress yourself until you feel you have reached a point beyond level 6. Then, while you continue to slowly stroke the same area of your genitals, switch your mental focus to another area of the genitals.

Men, if you reach just beyond level 6 by stroking the head of your penis, for example, continue stroking the head, but switch the focus of your attention to how the shaft of your penis feels.

Women, if you have reached just beyond level 6 by stroking your clitoris, continue stroking it, but switch your focus to the sensations in your inner vaginal lips.

After your arousal level has gone back down around to

about 5, switch your focus back to the area you are caressing until your arousal goes back up above 6. See if you can plateau at this level for thirty seconds or more by switching your focus from the sensation in one part of your genitals to another.

The basic technique is to focus on the area you are touching to allow your arousal level to go up, and switch your focus to an area that is not being touched to let your arousal level go down. Once you get the hang of doing it, switching your focus in this way will allow you to plateau at any level you choose.

The final technique you will use to plateau is squeezing the PC muscle. You have been exercising the PC muscle for some time now and it should be in good enough shape so that you can use it to help you plateau.

Plateauing Exercise #4 Begin with your genital self-caress and try to plateau at level 7 this time. Caress yourself slowly until you reach a point beyond 7. This may take some time. Just allow yourself to focus, breathe, and relax.

When you reach a point just past 7, squeeze your PC muscle a couple of times. This should take your arousal level down a bit each time you squeeze. When your arousal level goes below 6, caress yourself again until you get to 7. Then, squeeze your PC muscle to take your level down. Continue squeezing and allowing it to relax so that you can plateau at any level you wish for thirty seconds or more.

Men, when you use the PC muscle, you have to watch out that you squeeze just hard enough so that your arousal level goes down, but not so hard that this continuous squeezing makes your erection go down. It may take a little practice to know exactly how many squeezes to do and how hard to do them so that you affect your arousal but not your erection.

Now that you know four different techniques for plateauing, try combining them. With practice, you will be able to change your breathing, move your pelvis, switch your focus, and squeeze your PC muscle all at the same plateau. This is how you will be able to plateau at high levels for several minutes.

As I said before, it is important to learn each exercise one at a time. Try doing each exercise two to three times a week, until you feel really comfortable with it—then add a new one. I know they sound complicated, but with practice all of these techniques will become automatic and you won't have to think about them.

Once you have explored your body and become more aware of what pleases you and what affects your arousal, you are ready to move on to exercises that you and your partner do *together*.

Chapter Four

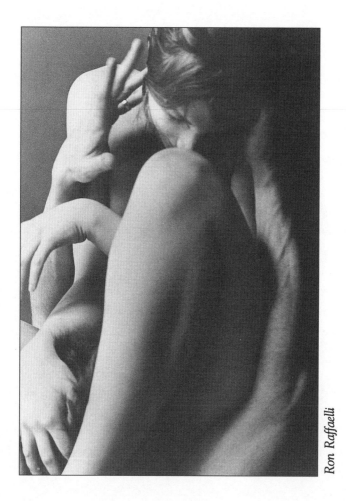

Ron Raffaelli

Partner Caresses That Kindle Desire

Now that you have taken the time to explore your sexuality with simple self-caresses, it is time to experience your partner's body in a whole new way. These basic sensate focus caresses are delightfully relaxing and get you in just the right mood to explore your sensuality. That's why I'll have you do one or more of these caresses as a prelude to most of the advanced exercises ahead. You will find they really do ignite your desire, even if you don't exactly feel desirous when you begin the exercises.

Am I suggesting that you don't wait until "the moment is right" to do sensate focus exercises? Yes.

Most people operate under the myth that spontaneous sex is the best kind; the more of a surprise, the sweeter the interlude. Somehow, the idea of penciling a lovemaking session into your datebook, the way you would a business luncheon or a dentist's appointment, seems rather, well, crass.

If you feel this way, you probably assume you have to wait until you feel mutual desire to try one of these exercises with your partner. I would counsel you not to wait. Instead, make a date to do them when you both have time. My experience with clients has shown that if you schedule time for these exercises, over time your desire will actually increase, whereas, if you wait for the "right" time, it could be a very long wait! I don't mean to discount spontaneous sexual desire—spontaneous sex can be great. But the truth is, sex will become more frequent only if you make the time for it.

The series of caresses I introduce below can help. They stimulate desire, and that is a boon in this modern age, where the hectic pace of life can cause a temporary loss of interest in sex. (I use the term "interest" synonymously with "desire.") Believe it or not, poor time management is one of the most common causes of the loss of sexual desire. Fatigue, stress, and boredom also take their toll, making inhibited sexual desire one of the primary sexual complaints of our society. Fortunately, these are treatable conditions. I am assuming that your healthy sexual desire is what led you to buy this book. But if fatigue, stress, or plain boredom are an issue for you, the exercises in this chapter can bring your desire back.

What *is* sexual desire? No one has really pinned it down or defined it to my satisfaction. Yet, a lot of people are convinced they have problems with it. I'm not so sure. I think desire springs from our fundamental longing for union. It seems to involve a mental state of readiness, a certain enlivening of the body, and a focusing of our attention on what can answer that hunger. Yet, how we feel about ourselves, our partner, and the circumstances of our lives will make an enormous difference in whether we feel desirous—and desirable—or not.

Libido, or sex drive, is an aspect of sexual desire, but it does not account for all of it. Libido is the psychic energy we get from our basic biological urges. It is also a measure of how often the body feels ready to have an orgasm. Libido is at least partially affected by genetics. It can also be affected by the diet we eat, by depression, and by other chemical and hormonal changes. Like sexual desire, libido fluctuates. Nobody has the same sex drive all the time, nor do we always feel the same level of desire.

How Sensate Focus Exercises Stir up Desire

Remember how we talked about the importance of relaxation to sexual desire and arousal? The basic sensate focus exercises you are about to learn next activate the relaxation response. Try them, and you'll see how the slow, pleasurable touch can restore a deep sense of calm. But the benefits don't stop there.

Since the exercises are new to you, they will alleviate sexual boredom. Because you have to plan and schedule time to do them, you get accustomed to making sexual activity a high priority in your life. The exercises will also gradually increase your sexual arousal. Although sexual arousal and desire are not the same thing, they reinforce each other. Increased arousal leads to increased desire, which then leads to more arousal, and so on.

To do these exercises properly, remember the sensate focus principles I discussed in Chapter 1. First, remember to focus on the *sensations* you feel at the exact place where your skin meets your partner's. Second, try to keep your awareness in the *here and now*. If you let your mind drift off to the chores you have planned for later in the day, or the project due at work, your desire won't even have a chance. But if you allow yourself to focus, appreciation builds. When you can appreciate your sensual experience with a partner, your desire for that contact increases and your pleasure in it grows.

Finally, focus on *nondemand* interaction, a basic concept I explained in the first chapter. When you are the active partner, caress for your own pleasure. Don't aim for—or expect—any particular response from your partner. When you are the passive partner, allow yourself to follow the sensations and enjoy them, without feeling that you have to respond.

Exercise 10
The Face Caress

The first sensate focus exercise in this program is the face caress. It will really relax you. Like the back caress which follows, this is a short, nonsexual caress that can be used to make the transition to a new, more sexual exercise.

Before You Begin   To do the face caress, you will need some type of skin lotion that you and your partner like. Make sure that you both find the scent and the texture appealing. You will also need a quiet room where you will not be disturbed for one hour, and a clock or watch to time the exercise.

The person who will be active first sits up with his or her back against a headboard or wall, and a pillow on his or her lap. The passive partner lies between the active partner's legs, head on the pillow, face up. You can do this caress with clothes on, nude, or partially nude, whichever is more comfortable.

Active Partner   Slowly caress your partner's face. Cover the area from the top of the head to the collarbone. Caress for your own pleasure, using the sensate focus techniques you read about in Chapter 1. Caress as slowly as you can. Pay attention to the temperature, texture, and shape of your partner's face. Experiment with using all of your fingertips, the knuckle of just one finger, or circling leisurely with the back of your hand. Just remember that this is not a massage. If you were doing a massage, you would try to feel and manipulate muscles under the skin. In a caress, you are trying to increase skin sensations.

Focus on the exact point of contact. If your mind drifts off to something else, bring it back to the sensations in your hand.

Caress for fifteen to twenty minutes, covering your lover's forehead, cheeks, bridge of the nose, chin, neck, and ears. If you start to get bored or lose focus, slow your touch down to about half the speed it was before. Pay attention to the various contours of the face and the places where skin texture changes. How do the eyebrows feel beneath your fingertips, or the lips?

If you think your partner is starting to fall asleep, give him or her a light tap on the shoulder. If you feel any sexual arousal during this caress, even if it's only minor, take a deep breath and allow that arousal to spread throughout your body. Don't fight off any arousal, and don't try to force yourself to feel more than you are feeling.

Passive Partner   As your partner caresses you, pay attention to the exact point of contact, where the fingertips are touching your skin. Does it bring a sense of warmth or cause the muscles to relax? Is it a little ticklish or deeply comforting? If your mind drifts off to something else, consciously bring it back to sensations you are feeling at the place you are being touched. As long as the sensations of the caress are pleasurable, don't say anything to your partner. Give your partner feedback only if he or she is doing something that bothers you.

Remember this is a nondemand exercise—you should feel completely free to lie back and enjoy the caress without giving feedback. Just revel in the sense of comfort that comes from having your face lovingly stroked. And remember to relax all of your muscles. Stay passive and don't move around, sigh, groan, or do anything because you want your partner to feel he or she is doing a "good job."

Keep your PC muscle relaxed, too. If you feel any of your muscles tensing up, consciously try to relax them. If you feel any sexual arousal during this caress, take a deep breath, allowing the arousal to radiate throughout your body.

After one person has been active for fifteen to twenty minutes, switch roles for another fifteen to twenty minutes. After the caress is over, lie down and belly breathe together for another couple of minutes.

Having your face stroked is very comforting, isn't it? For some people, it provides a physical experience of nurturing they have not felt since childhood. Doing the face caress brings you back in touch with sensuality at its most basic, which is pure body gratification. Until you can return to this state of basic enjoyment of your body, full-blown eroticism is probably not possible.

Exercise 11
The Back Caress

The back caress introduces some new elements. Since you do it in the nude, it may stir arousal. This caress includes the whole back of the body from the shoulders to the feet. You touch the buttocks, but do not include the genitals. You can do this in bed, or on some other roomy comfortable surface.

Before You Begin   Find some baby powder. Set aside about forty minutes for this exercise. Each of you will take a twenty-minute turn as the active partner.

Active Partner   Sprinkle some baby powder on your partner's back, from the shoulders to the feet.

Put yourself in close body contact with your partner, lying right up next to him or her. Now, slowly caress each part of your partner's back including the shoulders, arms, back, buttocks, thighs, and calves. Again, this is not a massage of the back muscles. Your touch should be light.

Use one hand to caress the upper body. Then move to a new position when you are ready to caress the lower body. You could also sit comfortably and do the caress with both hands if you prefer. Don't try to do the caress in a massage position by leaning over your partner's body. You need to stay comfortable.

As you are touching, pay attention to what you feel at the end of your fingertips or the back of your hand or your palm. Notice how different parts of the back feel when you are stroking them with your palm rather than your fingertips. Take plenty of time to appreciate the slopes and the valleys of your partner's body, as the lower back becomes the buttocks, and the buttocks give way to the legs. Notice the direction in which the hair is growing down the legs and the arms. You may find it especially enjoyable to touch the back of the neck, the spine, and the thighs right beneath the buttocks.

If your mind wanders off while you are doing this, bring it back to where you are touching. If you get bored, close your eyes and slow your touch down to half the speed it was before. Remember to caress for your own pleasure, and don't worry about what your partner is thinking or feeling. If you feel any sexual arousal during this exercise, take a deep breath. This will allow the arousal to spread throughout your whole body.

If your partner falls asleep, give him or her a light tap on the shoulder. Don't let your partner miss out on the sensation.

If you feel your partner tensing up, give a light tap on the area that is tense.

At the end of the exercise, use your hair, breasts, or whole body to caress your partner for a couple of minutes. Then lie on top of your partner or right up next to him or her and hold yourself close for a minute to finish up. This will help you continue to feel connected.

Passive Partner   Lie comfortably on your stomach with your arms and legs slightly spread.

Relax and enjoy the caress. Focus on the exact point of contact. If your mind wanders off to something other than the caress, practice bringing it back. Keep your mind in the here and now. Let your partner know if he or she is doing anything that bothers you. Don't say anything to your partner unless something hurts or bothers you. If you feel sexual arousal during this caress, take a deep breath so that the arousal will spread. Don't try to fight off the arousal, and don't force yourself to become aroused.

Relax all of your muscles. If a particular muscle tenses up, your partner will tap it. This will remind you to relax it. Keep your PC muscle relaxed.

After you've gone through the exercise once, switch roles. Then lie together and breathe normally for a few minutes.

The way I usually do the back caress is to snuggle up against my partner and use my hand to reach as many parts of his back as I can. Then I change positions so I can reach his legs and feet. I usually use some type of body powder to do this caress. It increases the sensual arousal for me, because my hands tend to perspire, which makes my touch a little rough.

Speaking of arousal, don't cheat and touch your partner's genitals when you do this exercise. When you include parts of the body that are not in the exercise, you are jumping ahead to a future exercise, rather than staying in the here and now. You are also interfering with your ability to focus on sensations, which is the priority here. We want to make your skin come alive with sensations, so that your sexual experience is also *sensually* rich.

Exercise 12
The Front Caress

If you have been looking forward to touching the genitals, you'll get your turn in this exercise. For the reasons I mentioned above, however, please don't spend any more time on the genitals than you do on the rest of the body. In this caress, you explore the front of your lover's body, from the shoulders to the feet. Do this exercise in the nude.

For this caress, and the two that follow, first spend five to ten minutes doing the back caress as a focusing caress. This will help you both relax before the main exercise, and you can review and reinforce the basics of sensate focus before you try something new.

Before You Begin   Have baby powder, mineral oil, and a towel on hand. Allow twenty minutes for each partner.

Active Partner   Sprinkle some baby powder on your partner's body from the shoulders to the feet.

Choose a comfortable position in which you can maintain as much body contact as possible with your partner. Keep at least one hand on your partner at all times so you don't startle him or her with a sudden touch. Caress for your own pleasure. Don't worry about what your partner might be thinking or feeling. Slowly caress each area including the shoulders, chest, arms, stomach, abdomen, genitals, thighs, and calves. Focus on the exact point of contact. If your mind drifts off, bring it back to what you are feeling right here, right now. Experiment with different patterns of touching and see how sensual you can make your touch.

If you start to get bored, close your eyes and slow down your caress to about half the speed it was before.

As you reach your partner's feet, start moving your caress back up toward the genitals. When you reach the genitals, pour a little baby oil on your hand and caress the genitals for a few minutes. Then wipe the baby oil off with the towel and continue the caress back up to the shoulders.

In this, as in any sensate focus exercise, there is no right or wrong way to caress. If you are caressing the skin lightly, doing it for your own pleasure, and doing it in a slow, sensuous way, you are doing it right. If your partner starts to tense up, lightly tap the tensed muscle as a reminder to relax it. If you get aroused during this caress, take a deep breath to allow your arousal to spread.

Caress for about twenty minutes. At the end of the caress, use your hair, chest, or the whole front of your body to caress your partner. Then lie on top of or right beside your partner to end the exercise.

After holding each other for a minute or so, switch roles.

Because this exercise exposes the chest and genitals, it can make some people anxious. You can help your partner relax by slowing your touch, breathing deeply enough to set a rhythm for both of you, and lightly tracing large circles around your lover's abdomen. If your partner still cannot relax, you can switch to a back or face caress.

Passive Partner   Lie comfortably on your back with your arms and legs slightly spread. As your partner caresses you, focus on the exact point of contact. If your mind drifts off to something else, bring it back to the exact point of contact. Keep all of your muscles completely relaxed, including your PC muscle.

Tell your partner if she or he does something that bothers you; otherwise, don't say anything. If you feel any sexual arousal during this caress, just enjoy it. Take a deep breath to help the arousal spread throughout your whole body.

After you have switched roles and completed the exercise a second time, lie together for a few minutes and breathe from your belly.

Exercise 13
The Genital Caress

For this exercise you will need baby powder and a lubricant. Finding the one that is right for you can make this even more sensuous, so you might want to experiment. I suggest using either an oil-based lubricant, like a light vegetable oil, baby oil, or mineral oil, or a water-based lubricant such as K-Y jelly. You may want to test the oil elsewhere on your skin before you decide, because some people are allergic to mineral-based oils.

Set aside an hour to do it.

Before you start, you should become familiar with important areas of the male and female genitals. For the female genitals, you will need to locate the pubic mound, the clitoris, the clitoral hood, the outer vaginal lips, the inner vaginal lips, the perineum, and the vaginal opening. All of these structures are visible. If you can't locate something, please refer to the anatomical drawings in the appendix of this book. Later on, I'll tell you how to locate the Grafenberg spot (G spot), which is not visible. Because of the location, some women have difficulty reaching their G spot themselves.

For male anatomy, you need to know the following areas: penis, head (or glans) of the penis, frenulum, penile shaft, and scrotum. Again, if you are uncertain about any of these, check the appendix.

Once you know how to find these areas on *yourself*, take your partner on a tour of your genitals. If you are a woman, sit, spread your legs, and put some lubricant on the genital area. Show your partner your pubic mound, clitoris, clitoral hood, outer lips, inner lips, and perineum. Use a mirror if it helps you.

Then have your partner put some lubricant on his finger and insert it about an inch into your vagina. Squeeze your PC muscle to show your partner its location. Have your partner insert his finger all the way into your vagina and feel the texture of the vaginal walls.

To show your partner how to find your G spot, have him hold his hand palm up and insert his longest finger straight into the vagina. When the finger is inserted as far as it will go, have him hook it back toward himself, as if he wanted to point to the pubic mound from inside. The spot that he is touching that provides an intense pleasurable feeling for you is the G spot. To your partner, this area will feel a little rougher or more textured than the rest of the vagina. Have your partner slowly move his finger around on the G spot. He will feel it swell and start to pulse.

If you are a man, sit with your legs spread and put some lubricant on your hand. Show your partner the head and shaft of your penis. If you are uncircumcised, show her how to pull back your foreskin. Show her your testicles, perineum, and frenulum, the extremely sensitive area on the underside of the penis at the base of the head.

Now that you are both familiar with each other's anatomy, you are ready to start the genital caress.

Before You Begin   Do short back caresses of five to ten minutes for each partner. Set aside another forty minutes so you can take a twenty minute turn in each role.

Active Partner   Spend some time on a front caress. Remember to caress as slowly as you can. Caress for your own pleasure and not to turn your partner on. Let your focus follow your fingers or hand as they move along your partner's skin. If you get distracted, bring your mind back to the area you are touching. If you feel yourself becoming mechanical or staying in one spot too long, slow down and pay attention to the temperature of the skin in the genital area and the various textures. If you feel your partner tensing up, lightly tap the tense muscle as a sign to relax.

If your partner is a woman, use lots of lubrication and slowly move your fingers over her vaginal lips, perineum, and clitoris. Then slowly insert your finger in her vagina. Stroke the PC muscle and the vaginal walls.

Insert your finger a little deeper and gently stroke the G spot until it starts to swell and pulse. Notice how this pulsing feels against your finger.

Do the first part of this caress sitting next to your partner and stroking her from the side. Then move around and lie between your partner's legs so that you can see the areas as you caress them.

If your partner is a man, put some lubricant on your hand and slowly caress his penis and scrotum. It does not matter if your partner has an erection or not. If he gets so aroused he ejaculates, you can lovingly apply a warm towel to the areas where you and he are sticky, and continue the caress.

Passive Partner   Lie on your back with your legs slightly spread and close your eyes. Stay passive even if you become aroused. You may find that it is possible to go all the way to orgasm without responding.

Try to keep all of your muscles, including the PC muscle, as relaxed as possible. Focus on exactly what you are feeling. If your mind drifts off, bring it back to the point of contact. Give your lover feedback only if she or he is doing something that bothers you.

If you feel yourself getting aroused, take a deep breath. If you feel you might have an orgasm, go ahead. Don't fight it off, but don't try to force one either. If you don't feel aroused, don't worry about it. Many people actually experience this caress as sensual rather than sexual.

Each partner should spend twenty minutes caressing the other. Then lie together and breathe for a couple of minutes when you are done.

If you want, you can also set aside some time to talk about what you each liked before you switch roles. Each partner can describe one or two things that felt especially good. The passive partner can also ask for a new kind of touch, and guide the active partner's hand if that helps to show exactly what kind of touch is desired.

Safe Sex and Sensate Focus

The next caress requires oral-genital contact.

As you may know, this is a behavior that can put you at risk for AIDS. So can unprotected intercourse. Many of these sensate focus partner exercises include one or both.

Before you do any of them, I urge you and your partner to take the precaution of being tested for AIDS and other sexually-transmitted diseases. If your tests are negative, but you have any cause for doubt, use condoms for three months and then get tested again. Be aware that the virus can remain undetected for long periods of time.

One of the reasons why I have not incorporated safe sex practices into the sensate focus techniques is because I have written this book for committed couples, and am assuming that AIDS will not be an issue for you. The other reason is that sensate focus emphasizes feeling as much as possible, and condoms tend to desensitize the penis.

Please don't put yourself at risk. If there is any chance of infection, use a condom to practice these sensate focus partner exercises or wait until you and your partner have received a clean bill of health.

If you do choose to use a condom, for safety or contraceptive reasons, please do not make the mistake of lubricating the penis for part of an exercise, putting a condom on, and then having intercourse. The condom can easily slip off or even deteriorate.

Exercise 14
The Sensate Focus Approach to Oral Sex

After you have done the genital caress enough to become comfortable with it, you are ready to try oral sex in a sensate focus way. If you have little experience with oral sex you may not enjoy it right away. But I encourage you to try it. There are few things as enjoyable as doing a sensuous, nondemand oral caress. The tongue has a lot of nerve endings and you may find it fun to discover which parts of your tongue are most sensitive and receptive to certain tastes and textures.

The genital caress includes your lips and tongue as well as your fingers. Remember to explore freely and do only what makes *you* feel good. Think of sensate focus oral sex with your partner as simply using your tongue instead of your hand. The same instructions apply. In other words, do it slowly, focus on the touch, and do not pressure your partner to respond.

One problem that people sometimes have with this exercise is that they revert to their old way of having oral sex rather than trying it the sensate focus way. Many people hold their tongue and neck stiff when they do oral sex. For this caress, you should completely relax your lips, tongue, and neck and do the caress that way.

Women, it is a good idea to let your partner know at the outset whether you are comfortable with him ejaculating while his penis is in or near your mouth. The exercise may or may not bring him to the point of ejaculation, but you should still discuss this. As an option, you could stop the exercise before it gets to this point. You can always return to it later. Or, if it is agreeable to both of you, you can clean up the ejaculate and continue with the exercise. This will be your partner's call—some men feel uncomfortable with oral stimulation after they have ejaculated.

Before You Begin   Set aside an hour for your practice session. Start by exchanging back caresses.

Active Partner   Start with a caress on the front of your partner's body for a few minutes. Then focus on the genital area and caress the genitals with your hand for a few minutes.

Then, if you feel like it, lean over your partner and try to caress in the same way with your lips and tongue.

Do the caress for your own pleasure. Focus on exactly what you are feeling. Notice how concentrating on your own sensations makes you much more attentive to the little things: the little warm spots, the places where the skin is most delicate, the areas of extreme sensitivity. How does it all feel against your tongue?

If you drift off to something else, either bring your focus back to what you are doing or change to doing something that will keep your attention. Don't pressure your partner to become aroused or wonder what she or he is thinking or feeling. If you are feeling any performance pressure, stop the oral part of the caress and back up to a stage in which you felt more comfortable. If you feel your partner tensing up, lightly tap the tense muscle as a signal to relax. Continue for fifteen to twenty minutes before you switch roles.

Passive Partner   Lie on your back with your legs slightly spread and close your eyes. Keep all of your muscles, including the PC muscle, as relaxed as possible.

Pay attention to the sensations you are experiencing. If your mind drifts off, return the focus to your sensations as soon as you catch it. Let your partner know if she or he does anything that bothers you.

Each time you feel your arousal increase, take a deep breath and let it spread. If you become very aroused and even have an orgasm or ejaculation that's fine. Don't try to hold back your arousal, or force it to happen.

Finish the exercise with belly breathing after each person has had a turn.

The Benefits of These Basic Exercises

Don't be surprised by how much even these first basic exercises increase your general level of desire. In the first place, they work because they relax you. The nondemand philosophy removes any pressure that could interfere with your arousal. The newness of them makes them fun. The fact that you have to schedule them makes you manage your time better, so you get into the habit of setting aside and valuing time to be intimate.

Each of the new exercises in the chapters ahead will also increase your desire. If this is a clear goal for you and your partner, pay special attention to the advanced peaking exercises in the chapters ahead. The more you master this peaking process, the more you and your partner can share the pleasures of heightened arousal.

The path to sexual pleasure, and eventually ecstasy, has mutual and individual steps. Now that you have the basic sensate focus exercises for enhancing your sexuality, sensitivity, and enjoyment of physical touch, I will devote the next two sections to separate discussions of male and female sexuality. Each section is filled with gender-specific tips and exercises. Some of the exercises are for you to do alone; others are to be done with your partner. Try to alternate them so you do an exercise for increasing your capacity for arousal one night and your partner does one for increasing his or her arousal on another night. In this way, your mutual awareness grows and your discoveries are balanced.

If you and your partner are both reading this book, I suggest you each read the men and women's sections. For truly sensational sex, you need to understand and appreciate each other's physicality and arousal patterns as best you can. The aim is not to make you the world's greatest lover. (You don't need to be to experience the world's greatest sex.) But if you really want to enhance your sexual pleasure, you need to do it *together*.

In the final section of the book, Mutuality and Intimacy, you will come together again—with greater knowledge and sexual pleasure—to explore the emotional and ecstatic realms of sensational sexuality.

Part Two
Sexual Arousal and Men

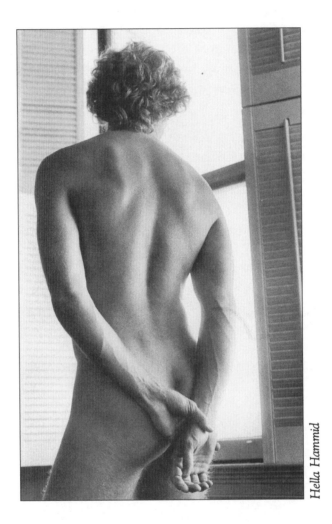

Hella Hammid

Chapter Five
The Male Sexual Pleasure Cycle

T he old cliché that "ignorance is bliss" does not apply to male sexuality. In fact, the keener a man's understanding of what is taking place in his genitals as he makes love, the more readily he can savor each step along the way. Even climax seems to last longer when a man really tunes in to these body processes.

Learning more about what's "normal" can also help a man relax and feel more confident in bed. Did you know, for instance, that arousal and erection do not always coincide? Or that erections do not always proceed upward in a straight line, but may cycle up and down? Or that it is possible to ejaculate without reaching orgasm or to experience an intense orgasm without ejaculating?

Men, the more you know about possible variations within the cycle, the more comfortable you'll be with your own sexual response cycle. That's why I've included the information below. Acquainting yourself with these facts will help you make the most of the exercises that follow to discover your full capacity for sexual delight. In the next three chapters, I share techniques for lasting longer, improving your erections, and enjoying ejaculation and orgasm.

Male Sexual Response

Based on their research and study, Masters and Johnson advanced the theory that sexual response proceeds in a series of stages—excitement, plateau, orgasm, and resolution. Each of these stages is accompanied by various body changes.

Their findings were based on laboratory studies of men and women volunteers who agreed to be monitored as they engaged in sexual activity. Masters and Johnson recorded heart rate, breathing rate, and blood pressure to figure out how the body changed as people became sexually aroused and reached orgasm.

They found that the **excitement** phase for men is usually accompanied by an erection, because excitement begins with blood flow to the genitals. At the **plateau** phase, they discovered, a man's erection becomes very firm and darker in color. He may secrete a few drops of clear liquid, a pre-seminal fluid produced by Cowper's glands, which are located at the base of the penis. (It is believed this fluid lubricates the urethra.)

Orgasm brings contractions of the long muscles of the body, as well as contractions of the pelvic muscles including the PC muscle. Blood pressure, heart rate, and breathing rate all reach a peak and then subside rapidly. Masters and Johnson thought that male orgasm always included ejaculation unless something was wrong. We now know this is not true.

During the **resolution** phase, the man's erection subsides and his body returns to its normal resting state. Most men experience a refractory period—some amount of time during which they cannot be stimulated further or have another erection or orgasm. A normal refractory period may last anywhere from several minutes to several hours.

Helen Singer Kaplan, another well-known sex therapist and researcher, added another phase to the sexual response cycle: the **desire** phase. This is a mental phase that precedes the excitement phase. During the desire phase a man thinks or fantasizes about sex or has some degree of interest in sexual activity.

New research has shown that actual male sexual response is different from this model in several important ways. For example, some men proceed through one excitement phase and one plateau phase. This does not mean that every man does so. Some men may have several plateaus prior to orgasm. Other men experience little or no refractory period.

Another fact that has been made clear since Masters and Johnson did their research is that male orgasm does not always include ejaculation. Some men are able to have an orgasm without ejaculating, and some men are able to have multiple orgasms. All of these responses are normal.

Based on this most current understanding, I have divided male sexual response into several different categories: desire, arousal, and erection. I will also describe the difference between orgasm and ejaculation. These processes are independent of each other, although they often go together. For example, some men mechanically have sex, maintain an erection, and ejaculate, but really feel little or no sense of desire.

What purpose is served by making these distinctions? My ultimate goal is to help you bring all of these pieces together. Lovemaking is much more thrilling when this occurs. The best way I know to do this is to acquaint you with each component of your sexual response. You may find one phase more pleasurable than another, or discover one that doesn't feel as great as you would like it to. Working with each component separately will help you concentrate your efforts where you choose, so that you can select the most appropriate exercises from the chapters that follow.

Sexual Desire

The sexual desire scale was developed by Helen Singer Kaplan. You may find it easier if you think of sexual desire in terms of how interested you are in having sex. If you have no interest in sexual activity and are rather bored, you would rate down at the bottom of the scale. But if your interest was so high you would rather be doing this activity than anything else, your interest would rate at the top of the scale.

You can see immediately that desire can be independent of both erection and arousal. It is possible to have a very hard erection and actually feel very little desire to have sex with your partner, whereas you could be having sex with your partner and have a very high desire level, yet lose your erection.

Sometimes psychological issues can interfere with desire. You may wish to consult a counselor if you think this is the case. However, if you simply want to enhance your desire, it's important that you and your partner make time for the basic focusing caresses in Chapter 4, or do the self-caresses and peaking and plateauing exercises in Chapter 3.

Arousal

Sexual arousal is a very important concept that I will explore in depth in the next three chapters. The arousal continuum ranges from a slight twinge feeling around your genitals up through orgasmic release.

Think of your sexual arousal as an internal process that is separate from your erection. Some signs of body arousal include rapid heartbeat, flushing of the face, shortness of breath, and a psychological sense of impending excitement.

Many men think that the presence of a drop or two of clear fluid at the tip of the penis means they are aroused. Yet,

Masters and Johnson saw this as an indication that a man had reached the plateau phase. In my experience with clients, sometimes this indicates a surge in arousal and sometimes it doesn't. Sometimes it can occur when a man is at a fairly low arousal level, and in some men this drop of fluid occurs when a man is not aroused at all. What this response actually indicates is that the PC muscle has spasmed involuntarily and forced this fluid out of the penis.

This book contains many exercises that will help you increase your arousal level. You will find most of them in Chapter 6, "Making the Pleasure Last and Last."

Erection

Erection is the filling of the penis with blood. You can have an erection without feeling aroused, or feel very aroused but not have an erection.

I usually describe erection as having four phases: initiation, filling, rigidity, and maintenance. **Initiation** is the mental mechanism that has to "let go" and tell you that it is okay to have an erection. This is an unconscious process—in most men erection is not under conscious control, but rather under the control of the autonomic nervous system.

Filling is the stage of erection in which blood begins to flow into the penis and the penis thickens. On a 1 to 10 scale, a 1 would be no erection, and levels 2, 3, and 4 would correspond to filling.

Erection is controlled by small valves in the blood circulation system at the base of the penis. **Rigidity** is achieved when enough blood has flowed into the penis so that the valves start to close off, trapping blood in the penis. The penis now has a "spring back" quality to it; if you push it down with your hand it will resist and become erect again. On the 1 to 10 scale, a 5 is the start of rigidity, and levels 6 through 10 indicate a progressively harder penis.

Rigidity is also described using the angle of the penis. For example, an erection that points straight up toward the navel is usually very hard, whereas an erection that points straight out is probably semi-hard.

The closing off of the valves at the base of the penis causes an erection to **maintain**, since the blood does not go in or out. It is normal, however, to get and lose an erection several times during the course of a sexual encounter. For some men, when direct stimulation of the penis stops, the erection may flag a bit. This does not mean that you have erection problems. It is also normal to feel your erections go up and down within a range of 6 to 10 during intercourse. Again, this does not indicate any erection problems, and is no cause for concern.

It is also normal to require direct stimulation, like fondling or kissing, before you become erect. I know that some men believe that if they are nude with a partner they find attractive, they should have an erection quickly, as in: "Two minutes have gone by—why don't I have an erection?"

The truth is that most men do not usually have an automatic erection just from being nude with a partner. So try to get rid of those internal timetables and experience your partner's touch without worrying about how long it takes you to become aroused or erect.

In general, a nice full erection creates a tight fit in your partner's vagina, and that means more sensation for both of you. Just be aware that a fully erect penis is not always the most enjoyable for your partner. I've found that most women prefer erections that are at a level 8. A fully erect or level 10 erection can be hard for the vagina to grip. There are some great exercises in Chapter 7, "Getting Better and Better (Erections) All the Time," for making your erections even stronger than they are now.

If you do have any problems with erections, you can save yourself an expensive trip to a urologist by comparing the erections you have with a partner with those you have in the morning. These morning erections are usually the hardest erections you have. In fact, if you have fairly hard erections in the morning but no erections with your partner, your problem is most likely the result of some kind of mental interference, which can be dealt with.

But let's say you don't have early morning or nighttime erections, *or* erections with your partner. Does this mean there is a medical cause for your erection problem? Not necessarily. Men sometimes temporarily lose their ability to have erections due to such factors as depression, fatigue, stress, or lack of sexual activity. So again the problem could have a psychological basis.

There are, of course, a number of medical conditions that can affect erections. Some of these include diabetes, endocrine problems, or circulatory problems such as hardening of the arteries. These are fairly rare as causes for erection problems, but men sometimes worry about these possibilities, and then develop erection problems that are psychological. Various drugs can affect erections, also. These include alcohol, nicotine and other stimulants, and some blood pressure, ulcer, antidepressant, and allergy medications. Men who have erection problems and suspect that an illness or drug is at fault should check with their physician.

Orgasm

When I talk about male orgasm, I am referring to something different from ejaculation. When you have an orgasm, the long muscles of your body, such as arms and legs, involuntarily contract. You experience a sudden steep rise in breathing and heart rate. What happens is that all of the muscular and autonomic tension builds to a peak and then is discharged quickly, giving you a feeling of release throughout your body.

Psychologically, orgasm feels like a very intense release. You also experience flushing of your face and neck, and an intense feeling of pleasure, like a hot light spreading throughout your body. Orgasm also includes muscular contractions of the internal pelvic organs such as the prostate gland.

Although any orgasm qualifies as a 10 on the arousal scale we have been using, some orgasms are more intense than others. For example, you may have an orgasm that includes only prostate contractions and a mild pleasurable feeling. Or, you may have an explosive orgasm that includes panting, moaning, tensing your face muscles, and full body contractions. All of these orgasmic responses are normal. The degree of intensity depends on a number of factors, such as how long it has been since your last orgasm.

Ejaculation

Ejaculation results when the PC muscle contracts, causing semen to be expelled from the penis. This does not always occur at the point of orgasm. Some men experience a sensational full body orgasm without an ejaculation. (Certain esoteric sects advocate this and claim it promotes longevity.) There are also men who ejaculate but experience no pleasurable or orgasmic sensations. Most men, however, do experience orgasm and ejaculation as one combined sensation. But it is possible to focus on them separately and appreciate each more, as you will learn in Chapter 8.

There are two separate phases of ejaculation: emission and expulsion. Learning to recognize these subtle differences during orgasm and ejaculation will make these moments of pleasure last much longer.

Emission, the first phase of ejaculation, occurs when semen begins to move from your vas deferens and prostate gland, where it is produced, and collects at the base of your penis. Psychologically, men experience this as the point of inevitability (POI). This is the feeling that an ejaculation has reached a stage where it is going to happen no matter what. Physically, you have a feeling of fullness at the base of the penis.

The second phase of ejaculation is **expulsion.** In this phase, your PC muscle starts to spasm and semen is expelled from your penis. If you pay close attention to your ejaculation you will be able to identify these two phases and feel how intense the pleasure is with each spurt of semen.

Keeping these phases in mind will help you with the exercises in the next three chapters. Remember, as you do them, how varied male sexual response is. Your arousal, erection, and orgasm patterns are probably normal, even if they do not correspond to Masters and Johnson's old four-phase blueprint. In sexuality there is a lot of room for the differences that make us all unique.

Chapter Six

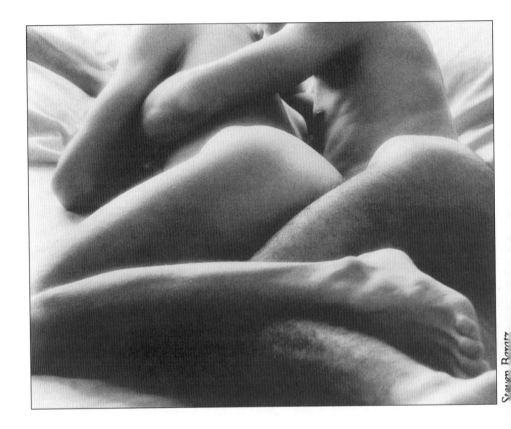

Steven Rosen

Making the Pleasure
Last and Last

W ould you like the experience of lasting as long as you want to, at deeply pleasurable levels of arousal? Have you ever wished to prolong lovemaking with your partner—but couldn't? These next set of exercises will heighten your capacity for pleasure. In a relaxed, pressure-free way, you learn the techniques and gradually gain the mastery you've always sensed was possible.

My male clients tell me these really work. *Tony's* comment is typical:

"Sometimes, I could last as long as I wanted to—other times, it seemed I'd ejaculate before I really got started. The exercises in this program made it predictable. There were no more surprises or disappointments."

Exercise 15
Arousal Awareness for Men

In Chapter 3 you learned to become aware of your arousal when you were caressing yourself. It was easy to pay attention to your arousal level when you had no distractions. Now you will learn to do the same while your lover fondles your penis and sensually explores you with her mouth and lips. This is going to be a little more challenging, but you are laying down a foundation that will serve you well when you have intercourse.

Remember that erection and arousal are two different processes, even though they often rise (or fall) together. In this exercise I want you to focus on your arousal, instead of your erection, and sense how close you are getting to orgasm and ejaculation. We will use the same 1 to 10 arousal scale I introduced you to in Chapter 3 to help you gauge your arousal.

As a quick review, a 1 is no arousal and a 10 is orgasm/ejaculation. A 2 or 3 is that slight twinge feeling at the base of the penis. A 4 is a steady, low level of arousal. A 5 or 6 is a medium level, and by the time you reach 7 or 8, you may feel your heart pounding, a flush on your face or chest, or some slight shortness of breath. A 9 is the point right before the point of inevitability.

As you and your partner do this exercise, I would like you to notice what happens to your arousal if you stay passive and allow yourself to experience pure pleasure with no pressure to perform. Remember to follow the basic sensate focus principles as you do this exercise and the ones that follow:

- when you are passive, focus on your sensations

- if your mind drifts off, bring it back to the exact point of contact between your skin and your partner's skin

- if your partner does anything that bothers you, let her know

- keep all your muscles relaxed

- remember to breathe

Before You Begin Exchange back caresses of about five to ten minutes each with your partner. Stimulate her with a front or genital caress before you begin the arousal awareness process.

The Exercise Lie on your back and take the passive role. Your partner begins a front caress and then a genital caress, during which she fondles your penis and scrotum. She can slowly move her fingers around the shaft and head of your penis and gently trace her fingers around each testicle. If she would like, she can then move into an oral caress, and use her tongue and lips to lick all over your penis, scrotum, and thighs. She should remember to explore for her own pleasure as she did in the early sensate focus exercises.

After a couple of minutes, your partner will ask you, "What is your arousal level now?" Tell her your level. If it is high, she will back off and allow your arousal to go down. If it is low, she will continue the caress.

Your partner can ask you your arousal level five times during a fifteen to twenty minute genital caress. Each time you tell your partner a level, take a deep breath and relax your pelvic muscles. Keep your PC muscle relaxed too.

Even though you are communicating with your partner, this is still a nondemand exercise. It doesn't matter how high you go or how short or long a time it takes to get there. If you are very aroused at the end of the exercise, tell your partner and ask her to help you reach an ejaculation and orgasm.

Exercise 16
Peaking for Men

The peaking process allows your arousal to proceed in a wave-like pattern that will help your brain secrete endorphins, those pleasure-giving chemicals that circulate throughout your body.

With each successive peak, more blood enters your penis, making you more and more aroused. The process will lead to a stronger orgasm and ejaculation.

This next set of exercises allows you to practice peaking first as the passive partner and then as the initiator. You need only do one of them per session.

Before You Begin Your partner will include hand and oral stimulation during this first peaking session. Make this a complete session, with relaxation exercises and focusing caresses for you both. Pleasure your partner with a front or genital caress.

The Exercise To start the peaking exercise, lie on your back and take the passive role. Your partner begins a slow front caress and gradually moves to the genitals.

Let her know when you reach level 3, either by saying "Three" or "Stop." Your partner then moves her hand to your belly, thighs, or some other part of your body until your arousal has dropped one or two levels. Then she will caress your genitals until you report a 4. She will stop and let your arousal go down again.

As you reach each peak, say the number level and then take a deep breath and relax your PC muscle and other pelvic muscles. Remember to stay passive throughout. Take a deep breath and relax your muscles whenever you feel a surge of arousal. If your partner notices you are tense or holding your breath, she can help you by reminding you to relax and breathe.

Continue peaking up through 5, 6, 7, 8, and 9, and all the way to ejaculation and orgasm at the final peak if you want to. Four or five peaks in any one twenty-minute session is enough, however.

Peaking Variation #1 You could do one session of peaking at only lower levels—2, 3, 4, and 5, and then the next session at higher levels—6, 7, 8, 9, and 10.

You could also do a session repeating the same level. For example, you could do a session with four peaks at level 7.

Stop between peaks long enough for your arousal to go down about two levels. It is just as important for you to get a sense that your arousal is going down as it is for you to get a sense of your arousal going up.

Repeat the peaking exercise as many times as you need to until you can easily reach 7 or 8 or until you can peak for about twenty minutes. Allow about five minutes for each complete up-and-down peak. If you want to have an orgasm and ejaculation at the end of a session, go ahead, but if you don't feel like it, don't force yourself.

Peaking Variation #2 You take the active role in this exercise. Begin it as you would any other, by exchanging back caresses with your partner. Then explore her body with a front or genital caress. When you are done, lie on your back and do any type of slow pelvic thrust or roll that you wish, as your partner strokes your genitals. Be sure not to tighten your stomach, thigh, or hip muscles.

Slowly thrust your penis against your partner's hand or mouth. When you reach a peak, tell your partner, stop moving, breathe, and relax your PC muscle. Continue for fifteen to twenty minutes. Take yourself as high as you would like.

When you're finished, pause a minute to take stock of how far you've come—from peaking by yourself, to peaking with your partner while you thrust. Appreciate your accomplishment.

Exercise 17
Male Peaking with Intercourse

Peaking can be done in any intercourse position. First, I would like you to try it with your lover on top, and you taking the passive role. Then, you can experiment with how peaking feels when you are the active partner.

Before You Begin   Start your session as usual with focusing caresses to relax yourselves and promote sensual arousal. Pleasure your partner with a front or genital caress, making sure she is lubricated enough and ready to take you inside of her.

The Exercise   Lie on your back and take the passive role. Have your partner do a front caress, a genital caress, and non-demand oral sex if she likes.

Peak up to a 4 and then to a 5 or 6. Be sure to allow enough time between peaks for your arousal to go down one or two levels. Notice how it feels when the blood recedes and then re-enters your penis.

Your partner will then climb on top of you and put your penis into her vagina. Remember to keep breathing as you feel yourself enter. She should start to move *very slowly*. Notice how wet she is, and how it feels to have her moving against you. Let her movements peak you up to progressively higher levels of arousal, even orgasm and ejaculation if you like. Be sure to allow about five minutes per peak so you are not rushing things.

Intercourse Peaking Variation #1   You can repeat this peaking exercise in a side-to-side intercourse position.

Peak with hand and oral stimulation to levels 4, 5, and 6. Then lie on your side facing your partner. Have her lie on her back with her legs interleaved with yours so that your genitals are up against each other.

Insert your penis and do pelvic rolls and thrusts to peak yourself up to 6, 7, 8, 9, and orgasm and ejaculation if you like.

After you are confident that you can peak in the side-to-side position or with your partner on top, use the following position in which you will control all movement and thrusting.

Intercourse Peaking Variation #2 You take the active role in this exercise. Before you begin, make sure you have your preferred lubrication handy. Then begin your session with relaxation and focusing caresses.

Peak up to 4, 5, and 6 with your partner doing manual and oral stimulation. Then do one or two comfortable peaks with your partner on top.

Have your partner lie on her back with a pillow under her buttocks. She should bend her knees, lift her legs up in the air, and spread them. (If she would like, she can rest her calves against her thighs.) This is a good time to apply lubrication to her vagina and your penis.

You kneel, sitting back on your heels, with your penis as close to your partner's vagina as possible. Support your body weight with your legs, not your arms.

Insert your penis and slowly begin to thrust. Move your penis in and out of the vagina by rolling or rocking your pelvis instead of tensing your thighs. Do this as slowly as you can.

Take five minutes per peak. At each peak, breathe deeply and relax your PC muscle and other pelvic muscles.

Remember to breathe evenly, focus on what it feels like to be inside her and move in ways that make you feel sensual. Think of yourself as caressing your partner's vagina with your penis. This will feel especially good as the peaking creates more fullness in your penis.

Peak yourself up to 6, 7, 8, 9, and orgasm and ejaculation if you wish. Notice how strong your orgasm is, as a result of practicing this series of peaking exercises.

Exercise 18
Using the PC Muscle to "Put on the Brakes"

Exercising your PC muscle every day, as I recommended in Chapter 3, will give you a good foundation for this next practice. Now you will use the PC muscle to help moderate your arousal.

Learning to use your PC muscle to "put the brakes on" your arousal is a little tricky. Normally, if you reach a certain level of arousal and then quickly squeeze the PC muscle once or twice, your arousal will go down a level. The reason this takes a little time to learn is that there are many different ways to squeeze. You may have to experiment a bit to see which works for you. It is best to work with this on your own first, before you try it with your partner.

Here are the basic types of PC muscle squeezes:

- one long hard squeeze

- two medium squeezes

- several quick squeezes in a row, similar to the way the PC muscle spasms during ejaculation

As you experiment, try to find the smallest amount of PC squeezing that you can do to take your arousal down a level without affecting your erection. If you squeeze your PC muscle too much before you have a full erection, you may temporarily lose your erection.

To find the best way to squeeze your PC muscle, do a peaking exercise by yourself as described in Chapter 3. At each peak, as you recognize the level, squeeze your PC muscle. Experiment with the different ways of squeezing to see which takes your arousal down a level but does not affect your erection.

The Exercise   Now you are ready to try using the PC squeeze in an exercise with your partner. Have your partner do a front and genital caress with you to start peaking. As you reach each peak, squeeze your PC muscle in your preferred way. Then tell your partner your level, breathe, and relax your muscles. Continue peaking and see if you can use your PC to lower your arousal even at level 9. Then allow yourself to have an orgasm and ejaculate if you wish.

Once you have learned to add the PC muscle into your arousal pattern, try using it with peaking in all of the intercourse positions I have described. Be careful, though, not to overuse the PC—do a peaking exercise without it once in a while. Overuse of your PC muscle can cause minor, temporary erection loss.

Exercise 19
Plateauing for Men

Once you have learned to use the PC muscle to peak, you can learn to plateau. Remember that plateauing is similar to peaking, except when you reach a desired level of arousal, you hold yourself at that level by fine-tuning your focusing, breathing, pelvic movements, and PC squeeze.

This next series of exercises allows you to experience plateauing with your partner. These really increase your staying power at very pleasurable levels of arousal. Do a separate one each session. Always remember to start with focusing caresses and to do a front or genital caress for your partner's pleasure so she doesn't feel left out.

Plateauing Exercise #1   For this first exercise, plateau at several different levels by using just the changes in your breathing. Plateau at each level for two to five minutes if you can.

To begin, lie on your back and your partner will do a front and genital caress, lovingly and slowly. Remember to relax, breathe, and focus on the areas where she is touching and licking.

As you reach a 4 on the arousal scale, try to stay there by changing your breathing. If you go beyond a 4, slow your breathing down until you are back at 4. If you go below a 4, speed up your breathing until you are slightly past a 4.

Plateauing Exercise #2 Try to plateau by doing pelvic rolls and thrusts instead of concentrating on your breathing. If you decide to plateau at 6, for example, start some pelvic movements at level 4. Roll sensuously, at various speeds. Then speed up the movements until you reach 6.

If you go beyond 6, slow your pelvic movements down until you are below a 6. Then speed up to allow your arousal to go up to 6 again.

Plateauing Exercise #3 Next, try to plateau by using your PC muscle to take your arousal down and pelvic movements to bring yourself back up. Soon you will be able to maintain your arousal level within a narrow range that you will control.

Plateauing Exercise #4 This technique involves switching your focus from one part of your body to another, or to a part of your partner's body.

For example, peak halfway to orgasm with some hand or oral stimulation from your partner. If you go beyond 6, switch your focus from the part of your penis that is being caressed to some other part. This will lower your arousal level. Then switch your focus back to the area being touched in order to move back up to 6.

Plateauing can be done with any kind of stimulation, including all of the intercourse positions. Soon you will find you can automatically hold yourself at any level of arousal you choose by making subtle shifts in your breathing, your focus, your pelvic movements, and your PC muscle. You will be able to plateau at level 9 or remain on the brink of orgasm for several seconds or even minutes.

Exercise 20
Repetitive Penetration

Many men can last as long as they want to with hand or oral stimulation but ejaculate sooner than they would like with intercourse. Sex therapists call this "point of penetration" anxiety. Whether this is a problem for you or not, this exercise will help you last longer with intercourse.

Before You Begin Exchange back caresses of about 10 minutes each and then do a front or genital caress with your partner. Make sure you have lubrication handy.

The Exercise Lie on your back and take the passive role. Have a couple of comfortable lower-level peaks as your partner sensually caresses you with her hands and lips.

Then change positions and have your partner lie on her back with her knees bent and her legs in the air. Apply lubrication to both of your hands. Kneel between your partner's legs and slowly begin to caress your penis with your hand, using a lot of lubrication.

With your other hand, caress your partner's genitals, also with a lot of lubrication. Then start to caress her genitals with your lubricated penis. Caress her outer genitals first and then insert just the head of your penis slowly into her vagina.

Remove your penis from her vagina and caress your partner's outer genitals with it again.

Then, insert your penis again and this time put most of it inside her vagina.

Practice several insertions within a fifteen-minute period, allowing yourself to go a little higher on the 1 to 10 arousal scale each time. Try to stay within the 4 to 8 range.

This can be a very erotic and satisfying exercise, and one you and your partner may wish to return to. You can relish each point of contact, and as you move deeper with each penetration your sexual pleasure will build exponentially.

Now that you have experienced the sensual gratification of lasting longer, I will give you some wonderful exercises that will make your erections even stronger and more satisfying.

Chapter Seven

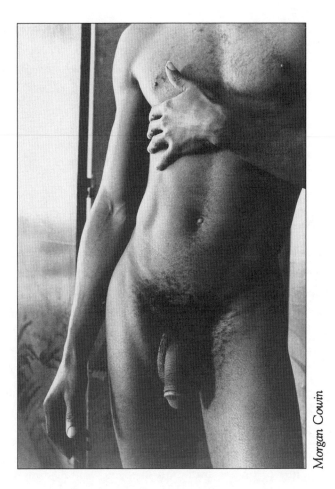

Morgan Cowin

Getting Better and Better
(Erections) All the Time

After you and your partner did the basic caress exercises in Chapter 4, you probably noticed firmer and longer erections right away. Get ready to see even more improvement as you try this next series of exercises. They really work, and they can be a lot of fun.

If you have any bad habits that prevent you from achieving really satisfying erections, these exercises can also help you overcome them.

I've included exercises that are specific to each of the distinct phases of erection. Remember from our earlier discussion that the phases of erection are initiation, filling, rigidity, and maintenance. Working with them separately will help you identify what your pleasure strengths are and where you could improve.

Just to review, **initiation** happens mentally when you give yourself "permission" to get an erection. **Filling** is the phase when the penis begins to fill with blood and appears to thicken. **Rigidity** occurs when the valves start to lock in blood so that the penis has a "spring back" quality. **Maintenance** is the ability to keep an erection for some length of time with or without stimulation. Some men are able to get a firm erection fairly quickly, but they lose it just as quickly. This is common in men over age fifty.

As I suggested earlier, if you want to know what your current capacity for rigidity is, try to observe the level of erection you get during the night, or when you first wake up in the morning. This morning erection is generally the strongest because it is entirely physiological. You are still asleep when it begins, so there are no thoughts to interfere with it. There is no anxiety, and little or no muscle tension to cause interference with the erection process.

Mental interference accounts for the fact that some men never get daytime erections as strong as their morning erections. Their daytime erections may reach only an 8 or 9 on the scale, even though their morning erections are clearly a 10.

The basic focusing caresses have probably caused you to experience some filling. While the size of your penis is no indicator of how much you and your partner will enjoy sex, it can enhance your mutual sexual pleasure to allow the fullness and hardness to increase. A fuller erection will give you the sense of being gripped by your partner's vagina, and excite her vagina by stretching it.

Erections that reach a hardness of about 8 are the most pleasurable for many women. If an erection is "too hard," however, the vaginal muscles seem to have a hard time gripping it.

Exercise 21

Priming the Penis for Quicker Erections

Here is a very effective exercise you can do by yourself to gradually increase your body's ability to generate an erection faster, with or without stimulation. The purpose of this exercise is to "prime" the system of blood vessels that helps you become erect by increasing your blood flow.

If you do this exercise for just five minutes every day, it will work whether you think it is working or not. Within two to three weeks, you will notice greater hardness in your morning erections and a general feeling of fullness in your penis during the day. You will also notice that it takes you less time to get an erection in sexually arousing situations with your partner. I have found this exercise very successful for men over 50, and those who have not been sexually active for some time and have concerns about how long it takes them to get an erection.

Before You Begin   Complete your daily PC muscle exercises first. Then, make sure you are relaxed. You could even do this exercise in the shower if you'd like. Make sure you have a lubricant handy.

The Exercise   Apply the lubricant to your hand, and slowly caress the base of your penis, squeezing the shaft and massaging the base. Do this *slowly*. Do not use a hard or fast masturbation stroke. You might try doing this with the hand other than the one you usually use during masturbation. If you are right-handed, for instance, use your left hand for this caress. It does not matter if you're aroused or not. Nor does it matter if you have an erection while you are doing this exercise. Continue caressing yourself for five minutes.

Exercise 22
Relaxing Your PC Muscle for Stronger Erections

Many men unconsciously tighten the PC muscle when they feel themselves starting to become erect. You develop this habit because at first, tightening it seems to pump up your erection. If you make a habit of this, however, you may start to notice after a while that it takes longer and longer to get an erection. If you react to this by squeezing harder, you will actually make matters worse. Here's why:

If you squeeze the PC muscle when you start to get an erection, your penis will fill a little bit momentarily because the blood flows in. After that, the temporary tightening of the muscle prevents more blood from flowing in to the penis, and the end result is a net loss. If you squeeze your PC muscle when your erection has already reached the stage of rigidity, however, your erection won't be affected, because no more blood could get in anyway.

Squeezing the PC muscle as you are getting an erection also works against your erection in two other ways. First, the sensation of tension actually travels along a feedback loop between your genitals and your brain. When your brain registers this "tension" message, it reacts in ways that interfere with your ability to feel the sensations of the first stages of erection.

Secondly, the fact that you are "doing something" to get an erection shifts you into a performance mode. This decreases your ability to relax and just allow your erection to happen.

Are you squeezing your PC muscle at an inopportune time? Try this exercise to see. Often, one session is all you need to break any bad habits. That may sound too good to be true, but I've seen it work this way with clients.

Before You Begin   Start the session with relaxation and focusing caresses. Then pleasure your partner with a nondemand genital caress.

The Exercise   Lie comfortably on your side or back in the passive role. Have your partner spend fifteen to twenty minutes slowly caressing your genitals with her hand and mouth. As you become aroused, if she feels you tighten your PC muscle, she will tell you and then wait for it to relax before she begins the caress again. After your partner has pointed out your unconscious tensing three or four times, you will begin to recognize it yourself, and so be able to keep your PC muscle relaxed without prompting.

You can allow yourself to go all the way to ejaculation during this caress if you want to.

Exercise 23
Synchronizing Your Arousal and Erection

For most men, erections increase as their arousal builds. Although these are separate processes, they generally appear to happen simultaneously. Men often have their hardest erections a few seconds before ejaculation. Sometimes, however, you may notice that your erection level lags a couple of points behind your arousal level. This usually isn't a problem, but sex does feel better when the two are in sync.

This partner exercise can help your erection level rise with your arousal. It allows you to practice alternating an erection peak with an arousal peak.

While you can't *will* your erection to become harder so that it matches your arousal level, you *can* manipulate your arousal level to sink until it matches your erection level. Arousal (which is psychological) goes down faster than erection does. As you do the exercise, you will find that each time your arousal level goes down to come into line with your erection level, the erection level—and your overall pleasure—will increase with your next peak.

Before You Begin Familiarize yourself with the 1 to 10 arousal scale you used in Chapter 3 and the 1 to 10 erection scale in Chapter 7. This time, you will switch back and forth between the two scales.

To begin, exchange some focusing caresses with your partner so that you are both relaxed. Then, pleasure her with a sensual caress.

The Exercise   Now lie on your back and shift into the passive role.

Have your partner caress your genitals with her hands or lips and tongue. If you approach arousal level 3 and you don't feel any erection filling, have your partner slow down so that your arousal level backs down to where your erection is. Then your partner can caress you again.

When you reach a filling stage erection (level 2–4), check your arousal level. If it is higher than your erection level, have your partner stop again so you can back down.

If you repeat this exercise a couple of times, you will notice that your erection and arousal levels tend to stay together, especially at the lower levels. You may want to repeat the exercise another couple of times to practice this technique at higher levels of arousal and erection.

Synchronizing Variation   You can also do this exercise during intercourse in which you are active.

Have your partner lie on her back, bend her knees, and lift her legs up in the air. Kneel in front of her and stroke her vaginal lips with your penis. Use plenty of lubrication.

As you caress the outside of your partner's vagina with your penis, peak yourself up to an arousal level of 4. Then notice if your erection is a 4. If it is not, slow your stimulation down until your arousal and erection level match. Notice what it feels like to bring the two together.

Continue stroking either outside or inside her vagina, moving sensuously in a way that thrills you. Every time you feel that your arousal level is going beyond your erection level, slow down and allow your arousal level to match your erection level. Enjoy the stronger, fuller erection that develops and the power of your orgasm, if you have one.

Techniques for Erection Filling and Hardness

One of the best exercises you can do to promote both filling and rigidity in your erection is peaking, the same exercise I described in both Chapter 3 and in Chapter 6. Peaking is a process in which you allow your arousal level to go up and down while you receive stimulation from your partner.

Here's how peaking promotes fuller and harder erections: if you pay attention to your arousal level and your closeness to orgasm and ejaculation rather than your erection level, you take the performance pressure off yourself to have a rigid erection, so your erection will rise naturally with your arousal.

For peaking to help your erection level, try the peaking exercises in the previous chapter. After the exercise, you and your partner can discuss the erection levels you had at various stages during the peaking process.

Exercise 24
Regaining Your Erection

There are certain myths that stand in the way of getting and keeping strong erections and having fabulous intercourse. One of these is the idea that once you have an erection, it should stay at the same level of hardness during intercourse until you have an ejaculation and orgasm.

Actually, it is perfectly normal for erections to get harder or softer several times during the course of a sexual exchange. When some men feel their erection start to get softer, whether during intercourse or before, they often tense up—which of course guarantees that the erection will go down even more.

If you begin to feel your erection flagging, "working" to keep it up is the worst thing you can do. The best thing is to just let go and *enjoy* the sensations in your penis. Take a deep breath, focus on your lover's touch, and relax your muscles.

The following exercise will show you how to enjoy losing and regaining your erection.

Before You Begin   Start with focusing caresses. Then, pleasure your partner with a front or genital caress. Allow at least twenty minutes for the following exercise.

The Exercise   Lie on your back and take the passive role. Your partner will start a nondemand front caress, genital caress, and oral sex. As always, she should do the caress for her own pleasure. Ask her to notice whether you are staying relaxed and remembering to breathe.

Whenever you have a noticeable filling erection response, have your partner stop the caress and allow your erection to go back to a 1. Then she can start over and allow your erection to go up to a higher level.

Have her repeat this several times during a twenty-minute period, allowing you to go up to several different levels of filling and rigidity.

After getting and losing your erection a few times, you will find your erection will maintain itself even when your partner's stimulation stops. You will find yourself actually *unable* to lose the erection because you have done the exercise so well.

If you subscribe to the myth that an erection should stay at the same level of hardness all the way through, you may feel frustrated the first time you try this exercise. When you feel your partner stop the stimulation, you will probably find that your first impulse is to tense up and squeeze your PC muscle to try to cause an erection. Your partner can point this out to you and remind you to focus, breathe, and relax.

With each attempt to lose your erection, try to become more comfortable with the sensation that your erection is going down. You'll get better at breathing and relaxing, and your erection will naturally come back up, allowing you to continue sensation-filled lovemaking.

Flaccid Insertion

It is also a common belief that a man's erection must be rock-hard in order for him to have intercourse. Now that you know the difference between filling and rigidity, you can use the following exercise to show yourself how to enjoy the sweet pleasure of intercourse *without* an erection!

This exercise is usually called "flaccid insertion," but other names for it include "quiet vagina" and "stuffing." It may sound strange, but it actually feels quite wonderful.

Before You Begin Make sure you have lubrication on hand. Start with focusing caresses, then pleasure your partner with a front or genital caress.

The Exercise Get into a side-to-side intercourse position. Lie on your side facing your partner, as she lies on her back with one leg on top of yours and the other in between. This way your genitals will be right up against each other.

Put a lot of lubrication on your penis. Gently open your partner's vagina with your fingers, and apply some lubrication. Take plenty of time with this and enjoy it.

You will get the best results if your penis is either flaccid or at some stage of filling (level 2, 3, or 4).

Have your partner gently fold your penis into her vagina, by pushing the base of your penis inside her. The head will naturally follow.

Once you are inside her vagina, breathe and relax your legs and your PC muscle. Notice how warm your partner's vagina is, and how wet it feels. See if you are aware of your erection level. Notice whether it changes.

You can keep your penis in her vagina without moving, or you can start to move and do one of the previous erection exercises inside the vagina.

Exercise 26
Oral Sex with the Man on Top

This exercise works really well for erection maintenance. Oral sex with the man on top is very stimulating, not only physically but psychologically. It's also good if you tend to get up to about a level 6 erection, and then are unable to go up any further.

Before You Begin   Start a peaking exercise in which you lie on your back and your partner caresses you. Pay attention to your arousal rather than your erection.

The Exercise   After you are able to do a couple of peaks at about arousal level 7, you will switch positions and have your partner lie on her back.

Get into a comfortable position either kneeling beside your partner or straddling her chest. Don't forget to focus and breathe, despite the excitement of this position.

Your partner will continue to peak you orally in this position by licking the underside of your penis and by putting your whole penis in her mouth, if she wishes.

You can also hold your penis in your hand and slowly caress your lover's mouth with it. Thrust into her mouth as slowly as you can.

The toughest thing about this exercise is getting comfortable in a kneeling position because you will be there for several minutes. Practice keeping your hips, thighs, and PC muscle as comfortable as possible. The more relaxed you are, the more receptive you'll be to the pleasurable sensations streaming through your penis as it is being licked and sucked.

Exercise 27
Repetitive Penetration for Erections

This exercise, which I introduced in the previous chapter, can help you achieve an even harder erection and maintain it during intercourse. When you do it this time, pay particular attention to your arousal level, rather than your erection level.

Before You Begin   Exchange focusing caresses and do a nondemand front or genital caress for your partner.

The Exercise   Start the peaking process by lying on your back. Have your partner take the active role and bring you to some low or medium arousal peaks.

Then switch positions and have your partner lie on her back with her knees bent and her legs up in the air. Put a lot of lubrication on both the penis and vagina and slowly caress the outside of your partner's vagina with your penis. Use this stimulation to peak yourself up to a 6, 7, and 8 on the *arousal* scale.

Next, insert the penis halfway into the vagina, do a peak, and withdraw until your arousal goes down two levels. Try another peak (about an 8) with your penis in her vagina and then withdraw again.

Repeat several peaks with withdrawal until you are confident you can penetrate with any level of erection. Notice how your penis doesn't have to be super-erect to penetrate her vagina. You are capable of doing the exercise no matter what level your erection is. Now try the same exercise but pay attention to the level of your arousal *and* your erection. You will find they keep getting better and better.

Repetitive Penetration Variation   In this exercise, you will "penetrate" various parts of your partner's body so that you start to think of her body as a sexual whole.

Begin with a front caress with your lover. Then caress her genitals with your fingers, lips, and tongue. Put lubrication on your penis (whether it is erect or not) and caress her body with it.

"Insert" your penis into your partner's armpit, elbow, knee joint, or any other opening you can create. Alternate these insertions with insertions into the vagina. Have fun with each other as you play around with this.

═══ **Exercise 28** ═══

Alternating Peaking with
Oral Sex and Intercourse

This exercise can help you maintain firmer erections during intercourse. You will alternate doing a peak with oral sex and then a peak during intercourse while kneeling over your partner. This is especially delicious because you get to experience both oral and vaginal stimulation.

Before You Begin   Exchange focusing caresses, then do a front or genital caress with your partner.

The Exercise   Start the peaking part of the exercise while you are lying on your back in the passive role.

Your partner can peak you up to low or medium levels of arousal with hand or oral stimulation. Then kneel beside your partner and have her peak you up to an 8 with oral sex. At that point, move around so you are kneeling between your partner's upraised legs and slowly do another peak up to an 8 with intercourse.

Then move back and do another peak with oral sex. At each peak remember to stop your movement, breathe, and relax your pelvic muscles.

Alternate oral peaks and intercourse peaks at high levels until you decide to ejaculate and have an orgasm.

Through the exercises in this chapter and the last, you have explored potent arousal, vigorous erections, and satisfying ejaculations. Now you will see how they can all work together so you can experience some of the best orgasms ever.

Chapter Eight

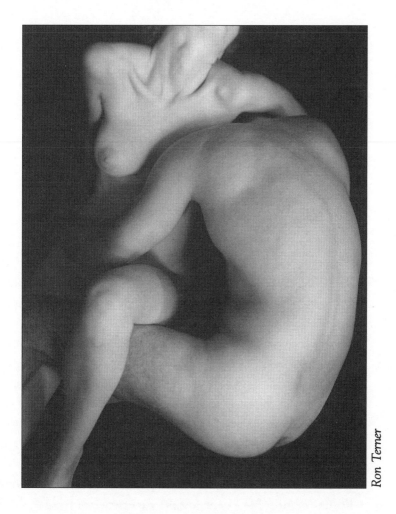

Ron Terner

Ejaculation and Orgasm:
From Ordinary to Extraordinary

I f you enjoy ejaculation and orgasm now, there are ways to make them even stronger and more powerful. Read through this chapter and see which techniques you would like to try first. The advanced orgasm and ejaculation exercises at the end of the chapter can have particularly potent effects.

It is not uncommon for adult men, over time, to begin to require intense stimulation of the penis before they can experience any sexual sensation at all. In sex therapy, the name for this condition is penile insensitivity. Over a period of time, if nothing is done about it, it can greatly interfere with a man's ability to have satisfying ejaculations when he is making love.

Fortunately, penile sensitivity can usually be restored. The exercises in this chapter can have positive results for *any* man within a month. My client *Joseph's* experience is typical:

"After years of having 'normal sex,' I found myself having difficulty ejaculating. Through these exercises, I learned to slow down, pay attention to how aroused I am, and relax my pelvic muscles so I could really enjoy ejaculation again."

Increasing Penile Sensitivity

One of the most common causes of decreased penile sensitivity is a man's masturbation style. You can masturbate in a way that actually decreases your sensations. This happens if the stroke is either too fast or applies too much pressure. After you have spent many years masturbating with a firm, hard stroke, you may not be able to feel a lighter, more sensitive touch with your lover.

Some men go long enough without having sex with a partner that they become unaccustomed to the delicate sensations of being inside a vagina. They "forget" how to enjoy feeling the inside of the vagina—caressing it with their penis—or experience its different sensations. So they find it difficult to ejaculate with just the stimulation of intercourse.

I've included these next few exercises for those of you who would like to change your masturbation habits to increase your sensitivity. All of them are exercises for you to do alone, and you should practice them two to three times a week. You may feel your sensitivity sharpen significantly in as little as a week, but it will probably take a month or so before you notice substantial change.

Decreasing Masturbation Time

How long do you usually take when you masturbate? Research indicates that some men masturbate to ejaculation in a few seconds, while others may spend several hours stimulating themselves before allowing themselves to ejaculate.

There is no "right" amount of time to spend before ejaculation. However, other sex therapists and I have found that clients who have the most penile sensitivity tend to spend about ten to fifteen minutes masturbating before they ejaculate.

If you currently like to masturbate for half an hour or more, there is nothing wrong with this. But keep in mind that this habit may cause your penis to be less sensitive than it could be. By reducing your masturbation time by half, you can increase your sensitivity a great deal.

The easiest way to do this is simply to keep track of how long you masturbate. You may be surprised to look at the clock and find you've gone on much longer than you thought. For two weeks, keep a chart of masturbation time. During week three, try to take five minutes off your time. Each successive week, try to take another five minutes off your time until you can easily masturbate to orgasm and ejaculation within ten minutes or so. This "tapering off" process will be much easier (and certainly more enjoyable) than trying to change your masturbation habits overnight.

Decreasing Frequency

Frequent masturbation also contributes to lowered penile sensitivity. There is no moral or health rule that says how much is "too much." However, cutting down on the frequency of masturbation can increase your sensitivity as well as "stockpile" your sexual energy.

Again, try keeping a two-week log to see how often you masturbate. Then, cut down the frequency by about 10 percent each subsequent week until you begin to feel a noticeable difference in your penile sensitivity and a greater ease and satisfaction in your ejaculations.

Some men find they can make all of these changes at the same time. You could keep track of your frequency *and* time over a two-week period, and then try to cut down on both. Then when you do masturbate, you could experiment with the next two exercises at least half of the time.

Other men find it easier to do this in stages. For example, they may decrease frequency first, then do a sensitivity exercise the next week, then decrease time the next week. Most of my clients have found that they reached their maximum sensitivity when they can easily masturbate to ejaculation within ten minutes while using a mostly-slow caressing stroke.

Exercise 29
Changing Your Stroke

Using an extremely firm, fast, high-pressure masturbation stroke is probably the most common cause of lowered penile sensitivity. It is difficult for me to describe what is too fast compared with a slow stroke, but this exercise will help you slow your stroke down and awaken your finer senses. Set aside fifteen to twenty minutes for it.

Begin masturbating with whatever stroke you usually use. Now slow down so you are stroking only about half as fast as you did before. After a minute, cut your speed in half again. Continue this slowing down until you are giving yourself a genital caress rather than masturbating.

Another way to change your stroke is to use your open palm or your fingertips and to caress your penis rather than using a closed fist to manipulate it. See if you can go slowly enough and use a light enough touch to feel which parts of your penis are more sensitive and which parts are less so. How delicate can you be? This caress should be similar to the genital caress described in Chapter 4. If you find it difficult to stay aroused with such a slow touch, alternate the old, firm stroke with the new, slower stroke.

Over a number of sessions your goal should be to spend most of your time with a slow, sensuous stroke. One way to do this is to keep track of, and gradually modify, the percentage of fast stroking and slow stroking you use each time you masturbate. You will increase your sensitivity if you can masturbate at least 80 percent of the time using a slow stroke. If you feel like ejaculating at the end of fifteen or twenty minutes, go ahead.

Exercise 30
Simulating the Vagina

Another way to change your masturbation habits is to find a way to masturbate that feels more like intercourse. Men have tried many creative ways to do this.

As I mentioned, some men are not fully gratified by intercourse because they are not used to being in a vagina. To simulate the feeling of a vagina, some men simply masturbate with one hand over the head of the penis and a lot of lubrication. Others masturbate into a reusable lambskin condom filled with a water-based lubricant. Still others use an empty banana peel heated up with hot water and filled with lubricant.

You can use anything you like that simulates the sensations of a vagina. Use your imagination and have fun with this. Find something that is well-lubricated, warm, and that can contain your penis.

Practice giving yourself a genital caress using your "vagina simulator" for fifteen or twenty minutes. Use the same slow, sensuous strokes you practiced in the previous exercise.

Advanced Orgasm and Ejaculation Exercises

If you would like to enhance your orgasmic potential even more, try the following more advanced exercises. Remember in Chapter 5 how I discussed the difference between orgasm and ejaculation, and described the two distinct phases of ejaculation? Learning to pay attention to these differences can result in a prolonged sense of exquisite pleasure.

Exercise 31
Prolonging Your Orgasm

Simply paying attention to your pelvic area at the moment of orgasm and ejaculation can result in a sense that your orgasmic response is longer. This exercise will also help you recognize your phases of ejaculation.

Before You Begin Start with focusing caresses to relax you both, and a nondemand front or genital caress for your partner.

The Exercise Start a long peaking process beginning with hand and oral stimulation. Then begin intercourse, with you as the active partner, on top.

Do several peaks and plateaus up to level 9 on the arousal scale. When you reach the point of inevitability, stop thrusting and take a deep breath. Feel the contractions of accessory organs such as your prostate, and then notice a few seconds later how your PC muscle starts to pulse. Breathe deeply, open your eyes wide, and focus all of your attention on the sensations in your genitals. You will distinctly feel each spurt of semen as you ejaculate, and will feel your orgasm and ejaculation sustained. Repeat this exercise until you are able to recognize all of these sensations.

Exercise 32
Using Your PC Muscle
to Strengthen Ejaculation

As soon as you are able to recognize the sensations of emission and expulsion, you can make your ejaculation stronger by squeezing the PC muscle at a particular point during sex. Do the exercise described above once more, but this time, when you reach the point right before the first involuntary PC muscle contraction hits, stop your movement, take a deep breath, open your eyes, and squeeze your PC muscle really hard! You will magnify your first PC contraction so that your ejaculation will feel as if it is exploding out of you. This can create an extremely intense orgasmic experience for both you and your partner.

The toughest part about this exercise is the timing. You need to practice Exercise 31 several times so that you can predict exactly when that first contraction is going to hit, and anticipate it for maximum pleasure.

Exercise 33
Enhancing Orgasmic Sensations

The two previous exercises dealt with enhancing your ejaculatory response. This one deals with enhancing your orgasmic response. Remember, ejaculation and orgasm are two different processes, although they often occur together.

To review, orgasm includes contractions of the long muscles of the body, increases in breathing, heart rate, and blood pressure, and a psychological sensation of intense release. The release is due to the fact that all of this muscular and autonomic tension and blood congestion in the genitals builds to a peak and then releases very suddenly.

The Exercise The first step toward enhancing your orgasmic sensations is to recognize them. So, do a peaking and plateauing session with intercourse and switch your focus to your breathing, heartbeat, and long muscle tension as you peak higher and higher. Stop your movement as you reach the point of inevitability and feel how all of this body tension dissipates after you ejaculate.

Next, do the exercise again and try to magnify either your breathing or your muscle tension. If you decide to change your breathing, as you reach a level 9 on the arousal scale, open your eyes and start to pant faster and faster. As you reach the point of inevitability, open your eyes and take several slow, deep breaths.

For your next session, as you peak up to level 9 with intercourse, periodically tighten and relax your arm and leg muscles as you thrust. As you reach the point of inevitability, tighten those muscles as hard as you can and then relax them as quickly as you can.

This might sound like it goes against the relaxation philosophy I have emphasized throughout this book, but *controlled* muscle tension can enhance your orgasmic experience if practiced at very high arousal levels. What you are doing is taking a response that your body has involuntarily during orgasm, and magnifying it to enhance the sensations. If you practice both of these responses (breathing and muscle tension), they will soon become natural and you will experience a stronger orgasm without having to pay attention to them.

■　　■　　■

As you worked through the exercises in this section, you sampled the great pleasures an explosive sensitivity can bring. Your stronger, prolonged erections and deeper arousal will excite not only you, but your lover, as well.

I encourage you to read the next section about female arousal and sensuality, and share in your partner's exercises. You will learn about the physiological areas of her arousal and discover together her emotional ones. This can be an enriching, sensual awakening for you both.

Once you and your lover get in touch with the sensuality and sexuality of your bodies, I also encourage you to explore the intimate, trust-building, and very erotic exercises in the last section of the book, Mutuality and Intimacy. Let them inspire your own erotic ideas, uncover deep facets of your sexuality, renew the playful aspects of lovemaking, and further your mutual path to ecstatic union.

Part Three
Sexual Arousal and Women

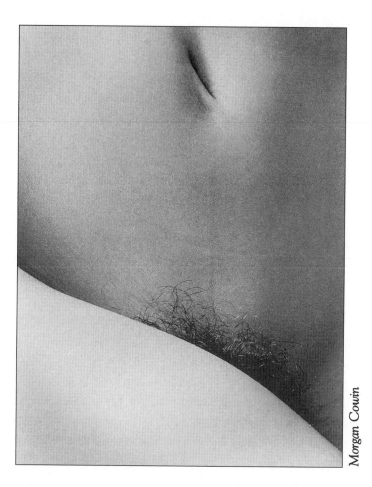

Morgan Cowin

Chapter Nine
The Female Sexual Pleasure Cycle

For a woman to awaken the full power of her sexuality, she needs to be on intimate terms with the six potential pleasure centers between her pubic bone in the front and her tailbone in the back. Only through exploration will she know which of these can bring her over the edge, and how to arouse them herself or through correctly positioning herself with her partner. She may also have to confront certain internalized attitudes that may hold her back from giving her sexuality full expression.

I will guide you through that territory below, and explain the advantages of certain intercourse positions. Men, you will also want to familiarize yourself with the intercourse positions that are most likely to provide the stimulation that lead your partner to orgasmic bliss.

The Female Sexual Response Cycle

What happens in a woman's body when she becomes aroused? Is the process significantly different from a man's arousal?

In some ways yes, and in some ways no.

A woman's sexual response—like a man's—also proceeds

through Helen Kaplan Singer's desire phase, and the four stages Masters and Johnson identified—excitement, plateau, orgasm, and resolution. Various body changes accompany each phase.

Blood flow accompanies arousal for women, as well as men. For men this is usually obvious—they get an erection. For women, arousal is not so obvious and mostly invisible. In fact, research has shown that women are not always aware that they are physiologically aroused. One reason for this may be that there are so many things going on in the female body during arousal that it is difficult to recognize any one change.

Here's what takes place:

During arousal, the erectile tissue within the clitoris fills with blood and the clitoris becomes hard. Both the inner and outer vaginal lips swell. The inner lips may actually turn dark pink or bright red. The body also produces vaginal lubrication, a fluid that comes out of the vaginal walls due to the pressure of the blood vessels in the musculature that surrounds these walls.

As a woman becomes more aroused, the middle section of her vagina may tighten and the inner third may open up. This is especially so if an object is inserted into the vagina. The muscles that support the uterus may tighten, causing the uterus to lift up. This causes the end of the vagina, the cul-de-sac, to open up.

It can be distracting to try to pay attention to any or all of these changes. That is why I suggest you use a simple 1 to 10 scale to describe your arousal, as we work to deepen it. I introduced you to this scale in Chapter 3 and we used it extensively in working with the men in the previous section. You will make use of it again in the following chapters as you learn to become more familiar with your arousal process and experiment with new ways to bring yourself to orgasm.

On the 1 to 10 arousal scale, orgasm is a 10. But, before I describe what happens when you have an orgasm, I want to

discuss some general issues and debunk some common misun-
derstandings about female orgasm.

Female Orgasm

There has been some controversy in the past about how women
have orgasms or even whether they have them at all. According to early psychoanalysts such as Sigmund Freud, orgasms
resulting from stimulation of the clitoris were in some way less
"mature" than orgasms originating in the vagina. Later the research conducted by Masters and Johnson indicated that all
female orgasms resulted from clitoral stimulation and there was
no such thing as a vaginal orgasm.

Then information started to come out about the G spot
and it became clear that there is at least one area within the
vagina where an orgasm can be triggered. So the old "clitoral
versus vaginal orgasm" debate became somewhat meaningless.

More recent research indicates that there are a *number* of
ways in which women have orgasms. Clitoral stimulation com-
monly produces orgasm, but some women experience orgasm
with no physical stimulation at all; for example, you may
awaken from an erotic dream and find you are having an orgasm. Others may experience orgasm through fondling their
breasts, especially the nipples.

We now know that there are a number of areas both inside and outside the vagina which can trigger orgasm. These are
the PC muscle, the G spot, the cul-de-sac, the cervix, and the
opening of the urethra. We consider the clitoris, the PC muscle, and the urethra "external" triggers, and the G spot, cul-de-
sac, and cervix "internal" triggers.

The Clitoris

The clitoris is considered an external female genital structure, even though it is located within the vulva. The clitoris contains erectile tissue, so that it protrudes and becomes hard when stimulated. Because of the erectile tissue, it is considered physiologically similar to the penis. As Masters and Johnson found, many women find it easiest to masturbate to orgasm using the clitoris as the site of stimulation.

The PC Muscle

You know from the early chapters that a well-toned PC muscle is important for pelvic health. Toning the muscle also makes arousal, penetration, and orgasm more satisfying. This is because strengthening the PC muscle tightens your vagina and builds muscle mass. The greater the muscle mass, the more blood can collect in that area. This increased blood flow adds to the sensations during arousal and creates a greater sense of release when the PC muscle spasms during orgasm, and the blood rushes back out. In fact, just stimulating the PC muscle can produce an orgasm. I'll explain how later in this section.

The Urethra

Research on females of other species indicates that stimulation at the opening of the urethra can trigger orgasm. Anecdotal evidence shows that many women also find stimulating the urethra very arousing, though it can also feel unpleasant. Sometimes this area is called the "U spot." (I know—this is getting to sound like the alphabet soup approach to female genitalia.)

The urethra is the very small external opening of the urinary tract through which you urinate. The best way to locate it is to push up on the clitoris and spread your vaginal lips with your fingers. If you wish to stimulate the opening of the urethra, do so gently because the urethra and bladder are very susceptible to irritation and infection. *Never* put objects in the urethra because they can get lodged in there.

The G Spot

I have also discussed the G spot, which is located on the upper wall of the vagina, about two-thirds of the way in. Have your partner help you find it, by inserting his longest finger into your vagina as far as it will go. Then have him hook the finger back toward himself. When he touches a spot that provides an intensely pleasurable feeling, he's found it. (You can try to find this spot yourself, but it is often difficult to do because it is hard to position your wrist just right.)

The G spot is an area of extreme sensitivity. Stimulating it often produces a very intense orgasmic response, which is sometimes accompanied by a female ejaculation or "gusher." A female ejaculation is the expulsion of a large amount of thin, clear fluid.

Many women have had this ejaculatory experience once and then never had it again. Some of them became afraid because they consulted a medical professional and were told that they had lost bladder control and urinated during intercourse. So, they never allowed themselves to let go and to have this intensely enjoyable experience again.

The fluid that is expelled during a G spot orgasm is definitely not urine. This fluid has been analyzed and it is composed of a substance that is similar to semen but without the sperm, like the fluid produced by the male prostate gland. The prostate gland is considered the closest male equivalent to the G spot.

The Cul-de-Sac

Most people are familiar with the clitoris and may have heard about the G spot by now. But the cul-de-sac is a new one for most women.

The vagina does not end at the cervix and uterus. When you are not aroused, the uterus rests on top of the vagina about two-thirds of the way back. When you become aroused, the muscles supporting the uterus tighten and the uterus lifts up, exposing an area of the vagina that normally is behind the cervix. This area is called the cul-de-sac, which comes from a French word meaning "bottom of the sack." It opens only when you are highly aroused.

The Cervix

The cervix is the knobby structure at the base of the uterus. You may also hear it referred to as the "neck" of the uterus. In some positions, the penis stimulates the cervix during intercourse. Some women experience this as an unpleasant cramping sensation, but for others, stimulation of the cervix can trigger an orgasm.

Changes During Orgasm

Despite the existence of so many body areas in which orgasms can be triggered, many women have never experienced one. Still others remain confused about what actually takes place when you have an orgasm, or what one feels like.

An orgasm feels like this: the muscles around your uterus and cervix spasm so that your abdomen sucks in, or it flutters. You may expel some air from your vagina. Your blood pressure, heart rate, and breathing all reach a peak. Your neck, arms, and legs may spasm involuntarily, and so does your PC muscle, moments later. You may feel a tingling sensation in some parts of your body, and a sensation of warmth that moves from your genitals up to your face, chest, and neck. All of the energy created by this is then rapidly discharged, and you experience a psychological feeling of release.

Orgasms vary in intensity from person to person, and even from orgasm to orgasm. Some orgasms may include only PC muscle spasms and a mild, good feeling. Others may be so strong they cause your body to arch off the bed. For research purposes, volunteers in sexuality labs are judged to have had an orgasm if the PC muscle spasms and heart rate peaks occur. I tell you all of this so you can take pressure off yourself about expecting your orgasm to occur in a particular way. Everyone is unique. What's important is that you open yourself more and more to your own orgasmic capacity, in whichever ways work best for you.

Using Intercourse Positions to Your Advantage

Some intercourse positions are more likely than others to provide the stimulation a woman needs to have an orgasm. This is because different positions stimulate different orgasm trigger areas. Here are the more common variations you and your partner should know about.

The female superior position, in which you straddle your partner, tends to stimulate the PC muscle, the G spot, the cervix, and the cul-de-sac. The rear entry position tends to stimulate the G spot and the cervix. The missionary position generally only stimulates to the PC muscle. The coital alignment technique, which I will describe in detail in an upcoming chapter, is an adjustment to the missionary position that allows stimulation of the clitoris to take place.

The intercourse position I recommend the most is a position in which the woman lies on her back with her knees bent and her legs up the air, and her partner kneels between her legs. The woman can rest her legs on his shoulders or, if she's flexible, she can rest her calves against her thighs. This position stimulates the PC muscle, the G spot, the cervix, and the cul-de-sac in the woman, and it allows her partner to easily withdraw his penis to use it to stimulate the clitoris and urethra. This position also allows for the deepest penetration by the man.

Of course, women find certain intercourse positions stimulating for reasons other than physiological ones. There are psychological factors at play, too. Some women simply prefer being face to face with their partners when they're making love. Others prefer the raw animal feeling of rear-entry vaginal intercourse. Knowing what turns you on—and off—emotionally is just as important as knowing what kind of physical stimulation you need.

Let's take a look now at some common concerns that keep women from bringing all of their aliveness to bed with them.

The Permission Factor

As my colleagues and I have noticed over the years, the psychological issues that can intrude on sensational sexuality seem to run along gender lines. For men, the biggies are penis size and performance fears. Women, on the other hand, seem to have difficulty giving themselves permission to *enjoy* their sensuality and their sexuality.

One reason for this is that unenlightened attitudes persist, even today. I still hear comments like the following, from clients as young as thirty: "I was told that only 'bad girls' enjoy sex," or "I was taught you have sex because it's your duty. I didn't know it was possible to enjoy it."

Another reason women hold back is poor body image. I know too many women who would rather skip sex because they feel fat and unattractive. As one client told me, "I don't feel okay about having sex because I don't feel comfortable about having my partner look at my body."

These attitudes are unfortunate. They keep you from owning your sexuality and coming to know yourself in the kind of depth that dispels such negative feelings. The sensate focus exercises in the chapters that follow can really transform your relationship with your body and your connection to it.

These are not the only issues, however, that can detract from your ability to fully experience pleasure when you are making love. I have identified the six that are most common for women. Let's look at each of them in detail.

Poor Body Image

Most women I talk to have a problem with their body image. Even the most beautiful women in the world find something to dislike about their own bodies. ·The reason is that we have become captive to a media-generated ideal that has little to do with reality. When you look at yourself in the mirror every day, consciously or unconsciously, you probably compare yourself with models, actresses, rock stars, socialites, and cheerleaders — all inhabitants of a fantasyland. Try to remember that the reflection that stares back at you is without the benefit of an image stylist, perfect lighting, and the right camera angles, not to mention the best plastic surgery and personal fitness trainers money can buy.

Don't allow a negative body image to stand in the way of your sexual enjoyment. Your partner likely appreciates your body the way it is and finds you very desirable. Women are much harder on themselves than their partners are. In surveys, men indicate that their standards of attractiveness are much more relaxed than women's. You may find your breasts or thighs unattractive, for instance, but chances are excellent that your partner likes the way they look and feel. In fact, anecdotal studies have shown that many men prefer their partners slightly heavier and softer than women would ideally like to be. To deny yourself sexual enjoyment because you think you don't meet certain standards of attractiveness is a waste. You can enjoy your sexuality and sensuality no matter what you think your body looks like—and your body will look better for it!

Of course, changes that make you feel better about yourself will help your sex life. Sex feels better when you are in good health. So, try to exercise moderately, quit smoking, and eat healthy foods. This will improve your skin tone and muscle tone—your overall fitness—and these do have a bearing on how much you enjoy sex. (This goes for men, too!) The exercises in Chapters 3 and 4 will help you learn to understand and appreciate your body's responses. Connecting with *all* your body's sensations will enrich your sensual and sexual ones.

Lack of Masturbation Experience

Another very common reason that women have difficulty enjoying sex is because they often have sex with a partner before they have explored their own bodies. Most men have masturbated for years before they ever have sex with a woman. But for many women, touching their own genitals has been taboo, and so they learned nothing about what stimulates and pleases them during lovemaking.

From clinical experience, I can tell you that the easiest clients to work with are those women who want to learn to have orgasms but have never masturbated. These women all do very well in therapy because their orgasm problem is a direct result of lack of education about their body and its responses. *Bonnie's* comments to me are typical of women in this situation:

"I had no idea of what my body was capable of," she said "I was always taught 'don't touch yourself *down there.*' The whole area was really the dark continent to me. I would feel things during intercourse but not have any idea what was causing those feelings. Now I know how to ask my partner for stimulation that I know will help me have an orgasm."

If you have never masturbated before, this self-stimulation

holds the key to sexual enjoyment for you. Use the self-caress-ing, peaking, and plateauing exercises in Chapter 4 and the exercises for female orgasms in an upcoming chapter to learn more about your own body without any performance pressure. Many of the exercises are designed to show you how to stimu-late your body in such a way that orgasm with intercourse will become easy. What you learn can make lovemaking even more blissful for you and your partner.

Performance Pressure

Feeling pressure to have an orgasm can make you tense during lovemaking. Sometimes, that pressure is internal. You put down yet another women's magazine article on how to have ten or-gasms in an hour and wonder, "Am I the only woman who can't have an orgasm during intercourse?" Your partner may compound the pressure by asking you, "Did you come?" when-ever you make love.

You may be relieved to learn that you have plenty of company. The inability to have an orgasm during intercourse is the most common sexual problem for women today. In fact, the scientific literature reveals that most women *don't* have orgasms during intercourse.

So which is it—everybody's having them, or nobody's having them? It doesn't matter, because *you* can have them! My experience has taught me that all women can have orgasms and have them during intercourse, if they do the exercises detailed later in this book, and receive the right kind of arousing touch.

Another source of performance pressure is the "seven min-ute myth." Research has shown that if a woman is going to have an orgasm during intercourse, it takes her an average of seven minutes. Unfortunately, most women have interpreted this to mean that if they haven't had an orgasm in seven min-utes, something is wrong with them. To make matters worse, men have interpreted this statement to mean, "The longer I can have intercourse, the more likely it is that my partner will have an orgasm."

Neither of these interpretations is correct. Some women will have an orgasm long after the "seven minutes" hits, and others will have one immediately upon penetration. Still others will not have an orgasm at all, regardless of how long intercourse lasts.

You are on your own timetable here and it doesn't matter how long you take to have an orgasm. The important thing to remember is to take the pressure off yourself. What matters is learning about your own body and accepting your unique arousal patterns. Then you can share this information with your partner and both benefit from it.

Lack of Assertiveness

Women are often shy about communicating their sexual needs or desires to their partner. Part of this is rooted in the old "nice girls don't do it, and they certainly don't *enjoy* it" myth—"If I don't mention it, maybe it isn't happening."

This is an attitude that is destined for the dustheap. It is up to you to take full responsibility for your own enjoyment, and this, of course, requires you to tell your partner what you like and don't like. If communicating with your partner about sexual issues is difficult for you now, you will find exercises in Chapter 12, "Strengthening the Bonds That Sustain You," that can make it easier. They show you how to give your partner feedback in a very structured way, in order to minimize any discomfort you may feel.

Sexual Abuse

Sexual abuse as a child or adolescent, or a sexual trauma as an adult, can have some very serious consequences for your sexual comfort and enjoyment.

It is common for those who have been sexually abused as

children to become afraid of sex or, conversely, to become quite promiscuous. These women shut down their feelings so they won't be hurt again. They feel betrayed, powerless, mistrustful, and out of control regarding sexuality.

If you have been sexually abused, you may need to see a counselor to help you recover from it and move beyond the experience to enjoy a full sexual life. You may find that the exercises described in this book, especially in Chapters 4 and 12, can help you rebuild your sexuality from the ground up— particularly if you have a loving partner you can share them with. You may have to take it slowly to learn about sex in a nontraumatic way.

Intrusive Thoughts

Men and women think differently. This comes as no surprise to anyone. There are a number of research findings regarding the different ways men and women process information.

Men seem to have an easier time compartmentalizing— that is, they seem to be more able to experience one thing at a time and tune out everything else, whereas women tend to have intrusive thoughts. This becomes very apparent in our sexuality. Women have a much more difficult time than men clearing the details of the day from their heads to free them-selves for sex. Then when they have sex, thoughts or worries about the day still intrude.

Men seem to have the opposite problem. They deny that anything else could be on their minds, and go ahead and try to have sex. This is one reason men experience the performance problems that they do.

Neither way of thinking is good. There must be a happy medium, in which you can clear your mind to allow yourself to focus on sex, but can accept your feelings enough to know that something is bothering you. Again, the sensate focus exercises described in Chapters 3 and 4 will help.

Fear of Letting Go

It is very common for women to feel inhibited during sex and afraid to just relax and let go. This inhibition frequently prevents orgasm. A woman feels she will look funny or lose control if she allows herself to have an orgasm, so she allows herself to only go so far and is not able to experience a full release.

If this tends to be an issue for you, the relaxation principles in Chapter 2 will help. In the next chapter, the orgasm techniques will show you how to experience intense levels of arousal without self-consciousness or fear of losing control.

Now that you are more familiar with the physiology and psychology of female sexuality, let's move on to exercises that can help you *experience* your sexuality more deeply than you ever have before.

Chapter Ten

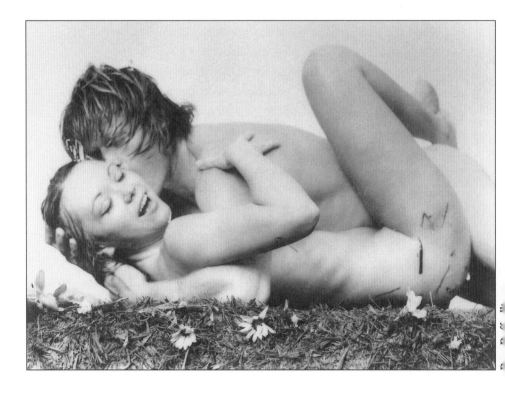

*Awakening Your Full
Capacity for Arousal*

Back in Chapter 3, I had you explore the nature of your own arousal, on your own, so you could come to know about this aspect of yourself in the most relaxed way. Now let's see how much more excitement you can create with your partner.

The five exercises that follow are similar to the ones I asked men to do in Chapter 6. Each of them can help to bring you to very deep levels of arousal. Some may even lead to orgasm. Don't pressure yourself to have one, but if you do, allow yourself to enjoy it fully. Deepening your arousal is a useful first step, whether you are orgasmic now or not.

Allow an hour for each of these exercises. You will take the passive role in each. Remember to follow the basic sensate focus principles, as you do them:

- when you are passive, focus on your sensations

- if your mind drifts off, bring it back to the exact point of contact between your skin and your partner's skin

- if your partner does anything that bothers you, let him know

- keep all your muscles relaxed

- remember to breathe

Begin each session with focusing caresses. Then pleasure your lover with a nondemand genital caress or an oral caress. What happens to your arousal as you stroke and lick him in the ways that you like best?

Exercise 34
Arousal Awareness for Women

Before You Begin   Review the arousal scale in Chapter 3. Set aside about twenty minutes for this part of the exercise.

The Exercise   Lie on your back comfortably with your arms and legs slightly spread.

Have your partner begin a front caress and gradually move to the genitals. He will then slowly do a genital caress, along with oral sex if he chooses to, in a very sensuous, slow, sensate focus manner. Pay attention to what you are sensing as his tongue strokes your vulva and your excitement builds.

Every five minutes or so, your partner will ask you your arousal level. Let your partner know what level you are at on the 1 to 10 arousal scale. Keep your focus on your mounting pleasure as he continues with the caress. Notice what feels particularly good.

Have your partner ask you about your arousal level four or five times during this twenty-minute exercise. It does not matter how high you go or whether your arousal level goes up or down when he asks. The important thing is for you to relax your body, recognize your levels of arousal, and communicate them to your partner.

The self-awareness you gain from this exercise is useful no matter how aroused it makes you. If it doesn't do much for you, tell your partner. But if it brings you to orgasm, go ahead and enjoy. Just don't push for it.

Exercise 35
Peaking for Women

The point of this exercise is to learn how to manipulate your arousal so that it starts to happen in a wave-like, predictable pattern. This will stimulate the release of endorphins, those feel-good chemicals that travel throughout your body. Fifteen or twenty minutes of peaking will build enough sexual energy to carry you to a sensational climax.

If your lover stimulates you in the ways I suggest, you may feel rapturous before the exercise is through.

Before You Begin   Locate some baby oil or your preferred body oil.

The Exercise   Lie comfortably on your back with your arms and legs slightly spread. Have your partner begin a front caress and gradually move to your genitals. He will caress these with oil, moving as slowly as possible, and will then spread your legs so he can see your inner vaginal lips.

Your partner will then slowly lick from the bottom of your vaginal opening up the center of your lips with the tip of his tongue. His tongue will glide or flick over your clitoris as if it were a "speed bump." Use all of your attention to follow the path his tongue takes. He should repeat this several times, each more slowly than the last. You may find this sensation quite thrilling.

He can also insert the tip of one finger into your vagina and stroke the muscles around your vaginal opening. You may feel the PC muscle spasm as it tightens around his finger.

When you reach a level 3 of arousal, tell your partner "Three." He will stop the caress for a few seconds to let your arousal go down a couple of levels. Really notice what happens in your body as your arousal drops. Then he will start caressing you again.

This time see if you can go up to level 5 and, if you can, let your partner know. You will be most likely to go up to the next arousal level if you remember to focus on your sensations, breathe, and keep all your muscles (including your PC muscle) relaxed.

With this continued manual and oral caressing, see if you can peak at levels, 6, 7, 8, and 9.

After each peak, let your arousal go back down about two levels.

If you reach orgasm during this exercise, that's fine. Try to stay as passive as you can during orgasm if it happens. Some amount of involuntary muscle tension usually occurs during orgasm, but the more passive you stay, the more familiar you will become with how your body feels during really high arousal levels and orgasm.

If you do not go up very high the first time you do this peaking exercise, don't worry about it. It sometimes takes some practice to be able to reach the higher levels. Recognizing your arousal level and telling your partner will help you go higher the next time. Remember that the sensations associated with the downcurve of a sexual peak are as important to recognize as the sensations that accompany the upcurve.

Repeat this exercise as many times as you and your partner like. Also, keep practicing peaking by yourself, as often as you like. Again, it will help you have stronger orgasms.

Exercise 36
Plateauing for Women

In this exercise you will learn to plateau, or maintain yourself at particular arousal levels with stimulation from your partner. Remember that breathing, using your PC muscle, pelvic movements, and switching your focus can help you maintain yourself at a particular arousal level. (To review these techniques, see Chapter 3.)

Another way to maintain your plateau is to ask your partner to stop and start stimulation. When you reach a point at which you would like to plateau, say "Stop." When your arousal starts to dip, say "Start." Or you can have your partner speed up and slow down the stimulation by saying "Faster" and "Slower."

Experiment to see how much sexual charge you can sustain. Notice how your body confidence builds as you become better and better at modulating your own arousal, riding the waves until you are ready to climax.

The Exercise   Lie on your back with your arms and legs slightly spread. Your partner will begin a front caress and then move to the genitals. Start by peaking up to 3 or 4 with some oral stimulation. When you reach a level 5, see if you can stay there for a few seconds by changing your breathing patterns. As you reach a level slightly higher than 5, slow your breathing down until you are back below 5.

Then to take yourself up above 5 again, breathe a little faster until you are almost panting. See if you can stay at level 5 for a few seconds or even minutes by just paying attention to your breathing and adjusting it. Next try a higher plateau by using your PC muscle to maintain your arousal level. As you reach a point slightly beyond 6, give your PC muscle a couple of squeezes until you are back below 6.

When you want to go to a higher arousal level, relax your PC muscle and let your arousal build. See if you can maintain your arousal level at about a 6 by just using your PC muscle.

Try plateaus at the same levels or higher levels using changes in your hip movements and in your focus. Notice which combination of techniques is most effective for you. Have your partner continue to caress your genitals using either his hand or his lips and tongue.

See if you can combine all of the plateauing techniques and use them at the same time. If you can plateau for a few seconds at level 7 or 8, you are ready to move on to the next exercises.

Exercise 37
Vaginal Peaking with a Partner

Women, practice this exercise until you are able to easily go up to level 8 during a twenty-minute period. Then you will be ready for the orgasm exercises in the next chapter. Your lover will be the active partner again.

The more you can focus *together* while your partner circles his penis slowly inside you, the more sensual this exercise will feel for both of you.

Before You Begin   Make sure you have a vaginal lubricant handy. You may actually have to start this exercise by providing your partner with some manual and oral stimulation so that he can become aroused enough to kneel over you and penetrate you. Usually a man can do the active part of this exercise even if he has a fairly low erection level.

The Exercise   Start with focusing caress, as you would any session. Then have your partner begin a front caress with you and move to the genitals.

With manual and oral stimulation, peak up to some comfortable levels like 3, 4, and 5. Now bend your legs and raise them in the air. You can leave them suspended or rest your calves against your thighs. Have your partner kneel between your legs with his genitals up against yours.

Your partner will then slowly rub his penis up against your vaginal lips, the same way he used his tongue during the previous peaking exercise. You will feel your clitoris as a bump that he slowly flicks with his penis. Peak at medium levels (5, 6, or 7) with this type of stimulation.

Both of you should remember to focus, breathe, and keep all of your muscles relaxed.

Then your partner will apply lubricant to your vagina and on his penis, before he begins to insert just the head of his penis into your vagina.

Do another peak while the head of his penis stimulates your PC muscle. Remember to breathe every time your arousal goes up.

Your partner will then insert his penis all the way into your vagina and go as slowly as he can. He should move it in a circular motion as well as in and out, focusing on his own sensations rather than trying to excite you.

Your partner will continue to slowly caress the inside of your vagina with his penis. Think of his penis as a giant tongue that is licking the inside of your vagina. If your partner's penis has a curve to it, see if you can feel it hitting your G spot. This may be so pleasurable that it takes your breath away, but remember to breathe.

You may find that you can peak at levels as high as 8 or 9 with this type of stimulation. If you are able to peak all the way to orgasm with this exercise, that's fine. Just enjoy it, especially if it happens several times. But be sure to peak at all those levels on the way up, too.

Exercise 38
Vaginal Plateauing with a Partner

This exercise will help you plateau during intercourse when your partner is active. Learning to plateau can help you have multiple orgasms. After you have one, ask your partner to keep exciting you so that your arousal level doesn't fall below a 9. At this point, it may only take a few strokes to bring you over the edge again.

Before You Begin   Make sure you've got lubricant handy. You may need to caress your partner before penetration so that he can become erect.

The Exercise   Lie on your back with your arms and legs slightly spread. Your partner will begin a front caress and will continue with a genital caress and some oral sex.

Do a couple of comfortable peaks at 3, 4, or 5. Then put your legs up in the air and bend your knees. Your partner will kneel between your legs and put lubrication on his penis and on your vagina. He will slowly start to caress your genitals with his penis. At first he will caress the outside of your genitals. Then he will slowly insert the head of his penis, and then the shaft until he is caressing the inside of you with his penis.

As your partner starts to stroke against you, see if you can plateau at 5, 6, 7, 8, or even 9 using the techniques you have practiced so far—breathing, PC muscle, hip movements, switching focus, and having your partner stop or start. Try combining techniques, or even use all of them at the same time.

For each plateau, tell your partner at what level you plan to plateau and how you plan to do it so that he will learn about your arousal patterns also. With practice, all of these techniques will become automatic and you will no longer need to think about them or plan them in order to do them.

Take about fifteen minutes to half an hour to do the penetration part of this exercise.

During this exercise, you can plateau at any levels you like. It is easiest to practice at the lower levels. This will help you to enjoy yourself more when you are ready to try plateauing at higher levels. Try to plateau at level 9 for as long as you can, and then just stop, and let yourself fall over into orgasm.

If you have done all the exercises in this chapter and would like to have even better orgasms, try the exercises in the next chapter. They will be very useful if you have not been able to have an orgasm during penetration.

Chapter Eleven

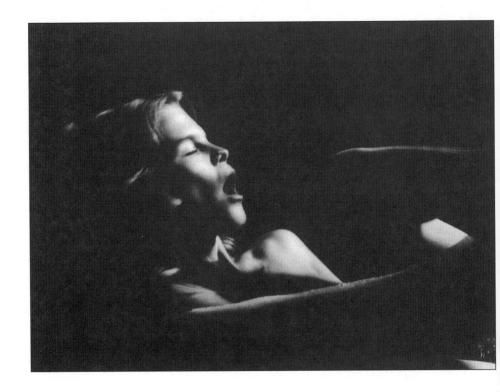

Sensate Focus Techniques
for Sensational Orgasms

I f you're orgasmic now, you'll love how this next set of
exercises can intensify your whole body pleasure in orgasm and show you brand new ways to bring yourself to
climax—once or several times in a row. If you aren't orgasmic
yet, I want you to know that I meant what I said a few chapters
back when I asserted that any woman can learn to reach orgasm with intercourse. If you're willing to commit to practicing
these exercises, and asking your partner for the right stimulation, you *will* see results.

You may even find that your dreams change! The more
often a woman has sex, and the more satisfying it is, and the
more likely she is to experience wild and wonderful climaxes in
her dreams.

Some of the exercises in this chapter are similar to the
ones in Chapter 8 that taught men how to enjoy orgasm and
ejaculation more. My philosophy is the same for men and
women—the better you know your own body and the easier
you have an orgasm with masturbation, the more satisfying your
orgasms when you make love to your partner.

In the first section of this chapter are exercises to enhance
orgasm with masturbation. Then you will move on to those
that can stimulate orgasm during intercourse. For best results,

do the solo exercises at least once a week, for the next two weeks. Then try to do the partner exercises one to three times a week, while you continue to do your own exercises as well.

Using Sexual Toys in Your Solo Explorations

The solo exercises below will make a big difference in how orgasmic you are when you have intercourse. Take care to pay attention to your response as you do them. If you have never experimented with sexual toys before, you will be surprised at how much they can help. My colleagues and I consistently recommend them to women who would like to learn to become more aroused and more orgasmic. I even hesitate to call them toys, because they do their job so well.

There are two types to choose from: vibrators and dildos. Dildos are always shaped like penises, while vibrators may or may not be.

Vibrators come in all shapes and sizes. Some are as small as car cigarette lighters, while others can be as large as your forearm. These larger vibrators are not meant to be inserted in the vagina and may have massage uses that are not necessarily sexual. Vibrators also differ in the strength of the stimulation they provide, depending on the battery size. Some contain more than one vibration setting.

Dildos do not necessarily vibrate. They also come in all sizes. They are usually meant to be inserted in the vagina. Some are made out of hard plastic, but the newer ones are made out of soft rubber or a gel-like substance that feels more like a real penis. Some are flexible and can be bent into different shapes. Some of the newer ones are made from molds of real penises, so they include details like realistic heads and veins. Some also include suction cups on the base so they can be freestanding.

If you purchase a dildo or vibrator to do these exercises, I recommend looking for one with the following features: First, make sure that it is shaped like a realistic penis and is about the size of your partner's penis. Second, look for one with a suction base. Third, make sure that it is also somewhat flexible so that it can be bent into a gooseneck shape to stimulate your G spot. And fourth, if you can get your full wish list, look for one that vibrates at both a high and low setting.

If you can find all of these qualities in one sexual aid, that's great. If not, you might need to buy two, for example: one with a gooseneck shape and one without.

Some of you may feel embarrassed about buying sexual aids like these. If you live in an urban area, you should be able to find a non-sleazy store that sells adult products and novelties. Alternately, you can order these products through the mail if you wish. An excellent mail order catalog featuring a variety of sexual toys and erotic products is "Good Vibrations," located in San Francisco. Call (415) 974-8990 to order a copy. Also, the back pages of popular magazines often have advertisements for companies that sell these products by mail.

Exercise 39
Using a Vibrator on Your Clitoris

This is the easiest female masturbation exercise, so we'll start with it. This exercise uses a vibrator to stimulate your clitoris, urethra, and vaginal lips. You will probably find that your clitoris is your most reliable orgasm trigger.

To use the vibrator effectively, hold it loosely and *gently* stimulate yourself. Don't make the mistake, as some women do, of holding the vibrator too tightly and pressing on your clitoris too firmly. If you hold it with the same level of tension you'd use to hold a pencil, you'll be fine. If you hold it any tighter, the stimulation will be too intense and you will find yourself fighting against it. Keep the stimulation on your clitoris or the area around it, which includes the urethral opening and the outer and inner lips. *Don't* insert it into your vagina.

I can't stress enough how important it is to pay attention to how you are using the vibrator. I once worked with a female client who was having difficulty with orgasm, and who complained to me that the vibrator wasn't helping her at all. I had her show me how she held the vibrator and how much pressure she used, demonstrating this on her hand. As we talked, I discovered she was doing a lot of things that prevented her from having an orgasm.

In addition to pressing the vibrator too hard against her clitoris, she was also using her vibrator on too high of a setting before she was aroused. She kept her leg muscles very tense and actually tensed up against the stimulation from the vibrator.

When she made the changes I recommended, she was able to become aroused enough to orgasm, both with and eventually without, a vibrator.

Before You Begin   Make sure your hands are clean and your fingernails are clean and trimmed.

The Exercise   Lie on your back and start a peaking and plateauing exercise by yourself. Remember to breathe, pay attention to your feelings, and stay relaxed—all basic sensate focus principles. Then start to stimulate your clitoris with your fingers. Do several peaks and plateaus with hand stimulation. Use the kind of touch that you know from experience excites you most.

Next, use the dildo without the vibrator to peak and plateau. Stimulate your clitoris, vaginal lips, and the opening of your urethra. If using the dildo is a new experience, notice *everything* about the way it feels against your body.

Now turn on the vibrator at a low setting and repeat the same peaks and plateaus. Again, if you've never used a vibrator, allow yourself to be curious about the sensations it creates.

Peak yourself up to several high levels with the vibrator. If possible, increase the vibration level as you peak higher. Peak yourself up to one orgasm or more if you would like. Don't hold back. You aren't limited to one. Be sure to adjust your breathing at the high arousal levels so that you are panting as you reach orgasm. Try some orgasms while staying passive. Then add in pelvic movements.

To maximize your orgasmic response, slowly and sensuously thrust against the vibrator as you use it to stimulate your clitoris. Do pelvic rolls and thrusts without tensing your thigh muscles.

Vibrator Variation   First, do some peaks and plateaus with the vibrator *before* you turn it on. Remember to breathe and to hold the vibrator loosely. Turn on the vibrator and slowly increase the stimulation to match your own arousal, not to force yourself to get aroused.

Do sensuous pelvic thrusts and rolls to respond to the stimulation of the vibrator. Notice what happens *throughout* your body as you move with the vibrator. Let the pulsation bring you to satiety.

This is the best way I know to use a vibrator to bring you to orgasm. You will discover the wonderful sensations your body responds to, which will also help you become orgasmic during intercourse.

Exercise 40
Vaginal Breathing

This exercise will help you identify the cul-de-sac and your uterine muscles. The contractions of your uterine muscles can greatly enhance your orgasm.

The cul-de-sac is the end of the vagina that normally remains closed off unless you are very aroused. When you become aroused, muscle tension causes the uterus to lift up and the cul-de-sac opens up.

Like any muscles, the ones that support your uterus respond to exercise. The problem is that many women find it difficult to exercise these muscles because they cannot identify them. The way to practice voluntary control of your uterine muscles is to practice sucking air into the vagina and blowing it back out.

The Exercise   Start by lying on your back and relaxing. Raise your knees, and experiment with tightening various muscles in your lower abdominal area. If tightening any of these muscle groups causes air to suck into your vagina, then you are using the correct muscles.

Practice sucking air in and out of your vagina. Your cul-de-sac is opening and closing every time you do this. After practicing solo, if you use these muscles during intercourse, it can have a deliciously pleasurable effect.

If you can't locate the right muscles lying flat on your back with your knees bent, try an old calisthenics position—the upside-down bicycling position. Do you remember this one from exercise class? You lie flat on your back and lift your lower body up by bracing yourself on your elbows. You don't need to actually 'bicycle.' The position alone will cause your uterus to settle on top of your vagina. When you return to a lying position, air will blow out of your vagina.

Practice alternating the bicycling position with lying down until you get a sense of which muscles are at work and then start to tighten them on your own to do the vaginal breathing exercise.

Exercise 41
Using a Dildo to Discover What You Like

This exercise, which uses a dildo, stimulates the PC muscle, the G spot, the cervix, and the cul-de-sac. It allows you to explore the orgasm trigger areas from the inside. The format is the same as in a peaking and plateauing exercise. Notice which triggers are the most pleasurable for you.

Before You Begin   If you don't remember how to find your G spot, refer back to page 120. Allow at least forty-five minutes to an hour for each session.

The Exercise   Lie on your back and start a self-caress. Start on the upper half of your body and gradually move to a genital caress using your hand. Then take your dildo and gently rub your clitoris. Peak at low levels with this type of stimulation.

Next, use your dildo to explore your vagina. Insert the dildo about one inch into the vagina and move it both in and out and in a circular motion. See if you can peak up to medium levels with this stimulation of the PC muscle. Then curve the dildo or switch to a curved one. Slowly insert the curved dildo straight into your vagina, and gently rub it against your G spot on the upper part of your vagina.

Feel the G spot start to swell and expand. Hook the dildo gently into the G spot and gently tug toward the opening of your vagina. Focus on the sensation this produces. Is it pleasurable, or too intense for you?

Now insert the dildo beyond the G spot into the end of the vagina. To find the cervix, move the dildo until you feel it rub against a knobby surface that yields a cramping sensation. Explore the cervix to find out how hard you can thrust against it or if you enjoy sensations in that area at all.

Now bend your legs and slowly thrust with the dildo as if you were having intercourse. At the same time, tighten your uterine muscles as you learned to do with vaginal breathing. Your cul-de-sac will open up and you will be able to insert your dildo into it. If you are very aroused when you do this, the feeling can be very intense, like plugging a cord into an electric socket. Notice whether you like this or not.

Now allow your cul-de-sac to close up with the dildo inside it. Gently pull on the dildo as you try to grip it. This is great exercise for your uterine muscles. With practice, you will be able to tighten your muscles so that you can tug really hard on the dildo without pulling it out. This can make you very adept at gripping your lover's penis during intercourse, which will delight your partner as much as it does you.

The first time you do this exercise, do it to explore the various areas inside the vagina. Then see if you can become so aware of the sensations inside your vagina that you can peak and plateau with this type of stimulation.

Dildo Variation #1   The next two exercises will prepare you to enjoy intercourse with your partner. If you can explore peaking and plateauing with a dildo, imagine how satisfying it will feel with your lover inside you.

For this exercise you will need a dildo with a suction base. You will be exploring the internal orgasm trigger sites such as the PC muscle, the G spot, the cervix, and the cul-de-sac, as you did above, but you'll use a different position.

To begin, lie on your back. Caress your upper and lower body using the sensate focus approach. Peak yourself up to medium levels of arousal with a genital caress. Then place the dildo's suction base on a flat surface, like the floor. Slowly kneel or squat on top of your dildo, and explore your PC muscle by moving up and down.

Then lower yourself more so that you can feel the dildo against your G spot. You may need to curve the head of the dildo to do this. See if you can stimulate your cervix, then suck in your uterine muscles and see if the cul-de-sac will open enough so you can fit the whole dildo into your vagina. Realize that it is more difficult to tighten your uterine muscles when you are kneeling or squatting than it is when you are lying on your back, so you may need extra practice to do this.

The first time you do this exercise, just use the dildo to explore the sensations that arise when you've touched one of your orgasm triggers. Don't pressure yourself to have to peak or plateau, because this will distract you from discovering what feels best. Then, when you are familiar with how these different areas respond to contact, thrust up and down on your dildo and do whatever peaks and plateaus you feel like.

Dildo Variation #2   This exercise is the best way I know to have a female ejaculation or "gusher" orgasm, which many women would like to experience but aren't sure how to acheive.

To begin, bend the tip of your dildo and place the suction area on a flat surface. Kneel or squat on top of your dildo and insert it so that you are stimulating your G spot. Gradually increase the pressure until you can feel your G spot start to swell and you become aroused up to about an 8.

Now change your position so you hook the curve of the dildo into your G spot. Thrust so that the dildo feels like a hook gently tugging at your G spot. Remember to breathe deeply and evenly to enhance your arousal.

At the moment of orgasm, climb off the dildo. You may experience a gushing of fluid down your legs. At the very least

you will experience a lot of lubrication—much more than normal. Keep practicing until you can have a "gusher."

Enjoying Orgasm with a Partner

You'll find these exercises similar to the ones in the last chapter, but this time *you* are the active partner. With these, you
can enjoy not only the physical but the psychological excitement of being the active lover.

Exercise 42
Peaking with Intercourse

Now that you have practiced a bit with toys and have already
done vaginal peaking with the man active, let's switch control
of the exercise to you.

When women do a peaking exercise, they have an advan-
tage over men, because they can peak to level 10—orgasm—
several times. Try for several really high peaks, each one focusing
on a different orgasm trigger. For example, try one whole set of
peaks in one position while you focus on the G spot. Then try
another set of peaks using your PC muscle as the focus of stimulation, then another using your cul-de-sac.

Before You Begin   Begin by lying next to your lover, and
exchange focusing caresses. Then pleasure him with a front,
genital, or oral caress.

The Exercise   When your partner has an erection, slowly
kneel on top of him and start to caress your genitals with his
penis in the same way he caressed you in the last chapter. He
should remain passive and relaxed.

Allow yourself to peak up to low and medium arousal levels (3, 4, 5, and 6) by caressing your vaginal lips and clitoris with his penis. Use his penis to pleasure yourself. Explore sensuously and spontaneously with different kinds of strokes. When you are ready to move on, insert just the head of his penis and stimulate your PC muscle. See if you can peak up to 7 doing this.

Remember to focus on your sensations, breathe, and keep your muscles as relaxed as possible even though you are kneeling. When you are ready, slowly lower yourself and insert his whole penis inside you. Move up and down on it as slowly as you wish. Use your partner's penis to explore your vagina the way you used your dildo. See if you can do a couple of peaks around level 8.

While you're at it, experiment with different ways to thrust. You can kneel so that you move straight up and down on your lover's penis. Use long thrusts and allow his penis to go all the way in and all the way out. Or you can squat over your partner if you have strong leg muscles. You may have practiced this with your suction-base dildo. You can rest part of your weight on the palms of your hands and use your arm strength to move yourself up and down on his penis.

Intercourse Peaking Variation #1   One of the most sensuous ways to do this exercise is to change your position slightly so that while you are still on top, you are thrusting back and forth on your partner's penis instead of up and down. To do this, kneel over him and lay against his chest. Support yourself on your elbows, and keep your buttocks as high in the air as possible while still keeping the penis inside of you. This will put the penis in contact with your G spot. You will be able to feel your partner's penis rubbing against the G spot as you slowly thrust back and forth. You may even have a "gusher."

Intercourse Peaking Variation #2   Try this exercise with pelvic thrusts, too. Think of yourself as thrusting up along the penis rather than down on it. Move your hips in a circular motion and slowly thrust your lover's penis all the way in and almost all the way out. Focus on every inch of it as it goes in and out. Go as slowly as possible, thinking of your vagina as a mouth sucking on the penis.

Peak to levels 7, 8, and 9, or do several peaks at level 9. At the moment before orgasm open your eyes, take a deep breath, and stop thrusting. Passively experience your orgasm— just allow it to happen. Feel your PC muscle spasm around the shaft of the penis. You will experience your orgasm as a shivering or spasming which may include not only your PC muscle, but your arms, legs, and facial muscles.

Exercise 43
Plateauing with Intercourse

Once you have learned to peak with your partner's penis, you can use the same positions and strokes to plateau at high arousal levels for long periods of time.

Before You Begin   Start with focusing caresses. Then pleasure your partner with a nondemand oral or genital caress. When he starts to get an erection, climb on top of him as you did in the previous exercise.

The Exercise   Do a couple of low level peaks (4 or 5) to get yourself used to the position.

Now try kneeling, squatting, or lying flat on your partner, as you call your plateauing skills into play. Remember that these include using your PC muscle, adjusting your breathing, changing your hip movements, and switching your focus. Practice plateauing at each orgasm trigger area using the techniques separately first, and then combining them until you can use all of them at the same time. Try to maintain yourself at higher arousal levels for longer periods of time. Practice as much of this as you can with your partner remaining passive. If he is focusing on the point of contact as you are, his arousal levels will rise as yours do. As you get better at this, your partner can start to move. If you have practiced plateauing at high levels with your partner passive, you will still be able to do it without being distracted by his movements.

Look at each other as you thrust. You can make this most exciting if you both focus *together* on your thrusting. That's even more important than how fast you thrust.

The best way to have an orgasm after a series of high plateaus is to plateau at level 9-plus using heavy breathing, intense pelvic thrusting, and PC muscle contractions. Then when you want to have an orgasm, stop everything you're doing. Just slam it to a halt—you will feel your body fall over into the orgasmic spasms involuntarily.

Exercise 44
Orgasm at the Moment of Penetration

Women have been taught that it takes from seven minutes to an hour to have an orgasm during intercourse. Actually, if you are not aroused, you won't have an orgasm regardless of how long intercourse lasts. But if you are *very* aroused, you can have an orgasm immediately upon penetration. *This really is possible.*

This exercise will show you how. The real secret to this exercise is peaking, not the penetration itself. You may need to spend fifteen to twenty minutes pleasuring yourself with your partner's penis. While you do this, it is important to remember the sensate focus principles and stay in the here and now. If you anticipate the orgasm or worry about it, it won't happen. Your ability to concentrate, peak yourself up to 9, and completely focus on that high level of arousal is what will produce the orgasm at the point of penetration.

Before You Begin   Start with focusing caresses. Then have your partner lie on his back, and lovingly stimulate him with a nondemand front and genital caress. As you do so, remember to focus on your sensations, touch for your own pleasure, breathe, and keep your muscles relaxed. Your partner should also focus on his sensations so he can fully enjoy the caress.

The Exercise   Start a nondemand oral genital caress. As your partner starts to get an erection, slowly stimulate yourself by rubbing his penis against your clitoris and vaginal lips, but don't insert it.

Peak up to levels 7 and 8 with this type of stimulation. In between your peaks, do oral sex with your partner so that he maintains high arousal levels. Peak up to level 9 by slowly rubbing his penis on your clitoris and outside your vagina.

Keep your leg muscles and PC muscle as relaxed as possible. Keep your eyes closed and increase your breathing. Then, when you are at the brink of orgasm, open your eyes, take a deep breath, and thrust yourself all the way down on his penis. You will likely have an orgasm, if not on the first stroke, then within about five strokes. Keep practicing this exercise until you can have an orgasm on the first stroke. If you peak yourself to level 9 several times before penetration, rather than only once, this will also increases your likelihood of having an immediate orgasm.

Penetration Orgasm Variation   You can use your PC muscle to help you have an orgasm on the first stroke. Do the exercise as described above, but when you sit on the penis, in addition to opening your eyes and taking a deep breath, slam your PC muscle shut around the shaft of the penis. This will often trigger an instant orgasm.

The CAT Position

This is a wonderful alternative to the missionary style of intercourse, which frankly, is the position least likely to bring a woman to climax. In the missionary position, the woman lies with her legs straight out and the man lies on top of her. In this position, it is difficult, if not impossible for a woman to move her pelvis. The only way she can thrust is to tense her leg muscles, and then the tension reduces her arousal.

There is a subtle adjustment you can make during missionary-position intercourse that provides more direct stimulation to the clitoris and greatly increases your chances of having an orgasm. This position is called the "coital alignment technique" or CAT. I have seen it bring arousal from a level 5 to a level 9.

Much of the research on this position was done by Edward Eichel and his colleagues. His research and the resulting techniques are described in his book, *The Perfect Fit*, which he wrote with Phillip Nobile.

Before You Begin   Exchange focusing caresses. Pleasure your partner with an oral or genital caress. Stimulate him until he has an erection.

The Exercise   When your partner has an erection, lie on your back. Your partner will lie flat on top of you and insert his penis as he normally would to have intercourse in the missionary position. Then—and this is the important adjustment to use the CAT—have your partner move his entire body up on top of you about two inches so that he is in the intercourse position once called "riding high." Your partner's pubic bone will rest on top of yours so that the base of his penis presses on your clitoris.

The type of thrusting you do with the CAT is different from the thrusting you may be used to. In normal thrusting, many couples like to move in opposite directions and actually slam their genitals together as thrusting becomes more vigorous. In the CAT position, both partners move together, and the actual range of movement is very small. It is as if your genitals are locked together and the clitoris and the base of the penis rub up against each other. Your pelvises will move but the rest of your bodies won't. The use of this position has many benefits. It will provide continuous stimulation of your clitoris during intercourse. And, since your bodies don't move that much, you are less likely to become fatigued. You can use this CAT position to do any peaking or plateauing exercise.

Exercise 46
Imitating Orgasm

If you have passively experienced the peaking process with your partner and tried the other orgasm exercises described in this book, chances are good that you have already had several orgasms. However, if you have not yet experienced orgasm, try this unusual twist: rather than faking an orgasm to please your partner, learn how to fake your body into thinking you are having an orgasm! This can actually trigger a real orgasm.

Remember that the orgasmic response is a full body response, not something that occurs only in your genitals. At the moment of orgasm, your face contorts, your arms, legs, and neck spasm, and your PC muscle contracts. This exercise is most likely to help you reach orgasm if you are able to peak up to level 9, but can't quite seem to go over the edge.

Before You Begin   You can do this exercise either by your-self with masturbation, or in any position with a partner. It may work best to do it at the end of a peaking or plateauing exercise. Or, you may want to begin with a focusing caress and then a genital caress.

The Exercise   Remember to focus, breathe, and relax. Stimulate yourself until you reach an arousal level of 9-plus. Then take a deep breath, suck in your lower abdomen, hunch your shoulders into the bed, thrust your pelvis up, open your eyes wide, and relax your PC muscle.

This may trigger an orgasm, which you will experience as a fluttering or spasming of the PC muscle.

I acknowledge that it's hard to remember all of the things to do at the same time. Practice each of them separately at higher and higher peaks or plateaus until you can do all of them together.

You can also pretend you are having an orgasm by acting the way you think highly orgasmic women act. Many of us believe that other women are wildly orgasmic in bed, but that we ourselves are repressed. You may think that other women out there respond sexually with screaming, moaning, and contortions, so if you act this way, you may be able to trigger your body to orgasm.

Another option is to wait until you are at the very brink of orgasm and then slam your PC muscle shut. This often results in orgasm.

Use these orgasm techniques not as ends in themselves but as ways to accustom yourself to having orgasms. As with any skill that involves learning complex patterns of behaviors and combining them, the first few tries will seem artificial. After you practice faking for a while, your body will "learn" what it feels like to orgasm, and eventually just staying focused and relaxed at level 9 will trigger orgasm.

■   ■   ■

As you explored the exercises in this section, you became more familiar with your body and gained an intimate awareness of its pleasure points and sensual potential. Are you now ready to indulge in the extraordinary sex this will spark?

Use your new-found body wisdom to savor the excitement that arises as your partner discovers his sexual potential in Part II, The Male Sexual Pleasure Response. Enjoy the sensations and intimate feelings that develop as you share in some of his explorations.

In the final section of this book, Mutuality and Intimacy, I give erotically-charged and playful ideas for building greater trust, intimacy, and sexual energy between you. The bonding and sense of connectedness you will feel with them offer an important starting place for explorations of mutual ecstasy.

Part Four
Mutuality and Intimacy

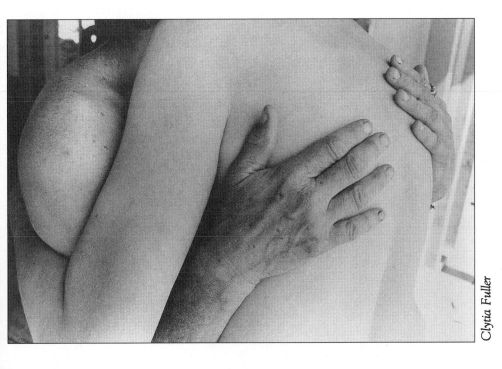

Clytia Fuller

Chapter Twelve
Strengthening the Bonds That Sustain You

If you have done the sensate focus exercises in the preceding chapters, you probably have a heightened sense of your own sexual aliveness and feel much more excited about being with your partner. As I have seen with client after client, doing these exercises together fosters deep intimacy. You create a bond through pleasure as you support each other in learning new skills. Trust—and appreciation—build as you follow through on your commitment to making your physical relationship better and better. This sensuous connection feeds your emotional life as a couple, as well.

In this chapter, I would like to give you some tools that specifically develop the emotional side of your relationship as you continue to grow physically close. It can be very scary to let down your guard enough to become more deeply intimate. Moving through the fear requires a lot of trust in your partner. The following practices are designed to help you build that trust, make it easier for you to communicate about what you like and don't like in bed, and draw out that spontaneous, playful part of you that remembers to keep sex fun.

Bonding provides a good foundation for these exercises because it offers a chance to feel close without pressure, and often creates a feeling of security. Let's start there.

Nonsexual Bonding

To "bond" is to form an emotional attachment with another person. Bonding typically refers to the emotional attachment that develops between a parent and child, especially during the first few hours of life. But adults also need to bond with their partners, in both nonsexual and sexual ways. It brings depth and richness to our relationships. Bonding makes us feel more secure and allows us to experience closeness in a pressure-free way. Nuzzling together is especially nice, particularly when you appreciate your partner's natural body scents or favorite colognes.

In this first exercise, you and your partner simply hold each other. I suggest you lie on your sides, face-to-face. Get comfortable, put your arms around each other and gaze into each other's eyes. Don't talk. Sometimes talking can enhance intimacy, but it can also create discord or distraction. We all need to spend to some time with our partner in which our bodies learn to know and trust each other on a physical level. Do this for about fifteen minutes—or longer if you like.

Here are other positions you can try later:

Spooning In this position, one person lies with their chest against their partner's back, and holds the other close by draping an arm over the other person's belly. This is not as intimate as the position you just used, because you are not face-to-face, but it is very relaxing because you can pay attention to each other's breathing. When you use this position, try to synchronize your breathing.

The Nurturing Position Lie on your sides again, facing each other. The partner in need of nurturing should slide down just low enough to burrow his or her face into the other's chest.

Lap Reclining One of you sits up in bed, on the couch, or even on the floor, and holds your lover as he or she reclines in your lap. This really helps you connect with each other again, especially after a long day or a period of separation.

I recommend at *least* five minutes of bonding a day. You can do it before you go to sleep at night, or in the morning when you both wake up. Choose your bonding position for each day based on how you feel. For example, if one of you had a bad day and needs to be nurtured, use the nurturing position. If you both need to relax, use the spoon position. If you feel pretty good and want to just be close, use the face-to-face eye-gaze position.

Sensual Kissing

In all this discussion of sexual pleasure, you may think I have ignored the simplest and easiest pleasure of all—a kiss. Well, I haven't. A kiss may be the most intimate, erotic caress you share with your lover. Some of our most sensitive nerve endings are in our lips, so it is no wonder that they can feel and communicate with exquisite precision. "A kiss can be a comma, a question mark, or an exclamation point," wrote Mistinguett. No wonder romance often begins with a kiss.

While sensual kissing, you kiss as you do any other sensate focus caress: kiss for your own pleasure, stay in the here and now, and focus on the exact point of contact—that velvety contact of your lips and tongues. Notice everything about your lover's kiss—the taste of her mouth, the feel of his tongue, the softness of your lips as they meet.

Gaze into each other's eyes and feel your connection. Focus, breathe, and relax, slowly licking your lover's mouth. You might graze your partner's lips or tongue with your teeth— whatever gives you various sensations of touch. The idea is not to leave each other's mouths sore, but rather to kiss as softly, seriously, sensually, and intimately as possible. Don't kiss too fast or too hard, and don't begin to think of where your kissing might lead. Just enjoy the moment.

Sensual kissing is a wonderful pleasure you and your lover can share leisurely or steal at a moment's notice. While it is a wonderful prelude to making love, it is important that you share it often outside of any other sexual contact. I suggest each partner give the other a kissing caress for at least five to ten minutes. Kissing can be the cornerstone of your sensual connection.

Sexual Bonding

I believe adults need to bond sexually with their partners, too. This happens naturally if you lie together, insert the penis into the vagina, wrap your arms around each other, and gaze into each other's eyes. Don't talk. Just look and appreciate.

Being physically close and connected at the genitals, without moving, and without any expectations, builds energy between you. Couples have reported feeling "bathed" in this energy which would otherwise be discharged by the movements of intercourse.

Try bonding in this way for about fifteen minutes and notice your experience. What does it feel like to just be inside her? How does it feel to have him so quietly inside you?

It doesn't matter if the man has an erection or not. If he does, fine. If the erection goes up and down, that's okay, too.

If he doesn't have an erection, he can lie on his side facing his partner. She can put lubrication on his penis and her vagina, and then lie on her back and interleave her legs with his. In this position, she'll find it easy to insert the penis, from the base first, as done in the "flaccid insertion" exercise in Chapter 7.

This does not have to lead to sexual intercourse. If you feel like it, after the fifteen minutes, go ahead. But don't feel pressured. Some people like to fall asleep this way, and others like to do this right after intercourse.

I recommend that you do this every day for five or ten minutes, as well. It is very powerful.

Sexual and nonsexual bonding, and sensuous kissing will create strong feelings of closeness between you. Few people take the time to do them, but it can really pay off in terms of enhanced intimacy.

Mutual Masturbation

Masturbation is one of the most intimate things that we do with ourselves. Many of us feel so intimate about it that we're hesitant to share this experience with a partner.

There are two ways to do this exercise. One way is to masturbate at the same time. Lie together on the bed, and stimulate yourself the same way you would if you were alone. Pay attention to your own arousal. If you want to, look at each other as you become more and more aroused while touching yourselves.

Or, you can take turns masturbating while the other watches. This is a very intimate thing to do, to share your most private activity with another person. After one person has masturbated for a few minutes, the other will take a turn. Try not to be self-conscious that your partner is watching you. Relax, close your eyes, and pleasure yourself the way you like to most. Take yourself as high as you would like.

This will help each of you learn how your partner likes to be touched. If you would like, you could try this with one partner cradling the other, while that person masturbates.

After you have done this together, talk about it. If it made you nervous or embarrassed in any way, share those feelings too. Telling each other the truth can only make you more intimate.

Share what you've learned about yourselves and from each other, doing this exercise.

Sharing Fantasies

Sharing your sexual fantasies as you masturbate together can deepen your intimacy. Decide who will go first. The active partner describes a fantasy while one or both of you masturbate.

If you're hesitant to share a fantasy because it's too revealing for your comfort, then create one in the moment about something you'd like to do to your present partner, or have done to you. Be lavish with the detail. Tell how it unfolds, how you feel, how your body responds. As you get more comfortable with this, you and your partner can share fantasies about other activities that you consider forbidden.

When you hear your partner's fantasy, try not to feel threatened. Accept that both you and your partner have sexual thoughts that may not concur, and realize that your partner is trying to be accepting of yours as well. Allow yourself to relax while you're listening, and appreciate the openness that your partner feels toward you to be sharing something so deeply personal.

Towel Over the Face

This exercise may sound very *un*-intimate at first. But it can truly build trust and banish performance pressure for both of you. *Bobbie's* experience was typical:

"The first time I tried it, it really freaked me out," she said. "I had so much going on mentally I wasn't even aware of what my partner was doing. But then I let myself relax. It was great to have no responsibility."

In this exercise, you place a light towel or piece of cloth-
ing over your lover's face. Then you pretend that your lover's
body is a toy that you can play with, for twenty minutes to an
hour. You can use any part of your partner's body to give yourself pleasure.

Your partner will also take a turn doing the same.

I recommend that the woman go first so that she is lubricated and ready when her partner takes his turn. It's also a good
idea to have vaginal lubrication on hand, just in case.

Pointers for Women   When you're the active one, slowly
rub yourself all over your partner. Lick his body. Masturbate
with his penis. Climb on top of his penis and slowly thrust in
and out. Masturbate by rubbing your clitoris on your partner's
knees or hips. Thrill yourself and moan appreciatively.

Remind yourself that sex is an animal activity. Feel free to
grunt, groan, bare your teeth, lightly nibble on your partner, or
growl as you are active during this exercise.

Pointers for Men   When you are active, pretend your
partner is a doll that you can play with for the next few minutes. Have you ever had a fantasy of having sex with a sleeping
woman? Now is the time to indulge that fantasy. Rub yourself
against her, rub your penis all over her, insert your penis into
her vagina. She will try her best to remain passive.

Pointers for the Passive Partner   Adjust the towel on
your face so you can breathe, but you cannot see.

Try not to move or respond in any way, unless your partner is doing something that hurts or bothers you. If so, tell him
or her.

It will be a little scary not to know what your lover is
going to do next. You may feel yourself tense up, but remind
yourself to relax. Explore what it feels like to have no responsibility for what happens. What it feels like to be "in" your

lover's fantasy. It's your lover's responsibility to make sure he or she has fun, not yours.

If you have an erection, an orgasm, or an ejaculation, just take a deep breath and enjoy yourself.

This exercise will help you trust that your partner is not going to do anything to hurt you. If you've done this and found that it increased your mutual trust, you may be ready for the next exercise. This one will really help you explore the limits of your trust with your partner.

Bondage

In this exercise, you'll let your partner gently tie up some part of your body or gently restrain you. Velcro or fur-lined restraints are available at adult stores or through catalogs. You can also use stockings or other items you have around the house.

Other than that, do this exercise just as you did the last one. Allow each partner a twenty-minute turn.

When you are active, tie up your partner. Then use your partner's body to pleasure yourself. When you are passive, tell your partner if she or he is doing anything that hurts you. If not, stay passive. Remember to remain aware that you have no responsibility at all in this situation. Relax as much as you can and focus on your sensations.

Many people are aroused by being tied up because it feels kinky and a little bit dangerous. You will become much more intimate doing this together and learning you can really trust each other.

"I was a little hesitant to try this, but I was curious, too," said my client *Susan*. "As I started to trust my partner, I could feel myself relax and stop fighting the feelings. The big difference between doing the exercise this way, and doing it as part of S & M, is that the turn-on in S & M is the fear in the tied-up partner as she or he fights against the bonds. That's not what happens here."

Drawing Close Through Better Communication

Good communication is as essential to intimacy as trust. Up until now, you have been developing your ability to communicate through touch. With few exceptions, the sensate focus exercises I have had you do were nonverbal.

There was a reason for this. I wanted you to feel as free from pressure as possible, while you were learning the basics. Getting you to stop talking also encourages you to *feel* more.

When you progressed to the peaking and plateauing exercises, you did share some very specific information with each other about your arousal levels. My intention here was to lay down a foundation for helpful communication, so you could overcome any negative communication habits you may have had. Many people think that they are good at sexual communication, when, in fact they come off as either whiny or demanding to their partners.

The way you communicate really can get in the way, as my client *Jack* discovered:

"I never realized before how my wife and I would say things during sex and the other person would take it the wrong way," he told me. "It seemed like if you said it during sex, even the most innocent comment would take on this huge meaning. These techniques showed me how to recognize what I was feeling and say it immediately. We are not reading as much negative stuff into simple comments anymore, so we have a lot more energy to devote to pleasure."

Genital Caressing
with Verbal Sharing

It's time to bring talk and touch back together. In these next five exercises, you will practice talking with each other about sex in a positive, self-affirming way.

Let's begin with a genital caress, where you give specific feedback about what you like after the touching stops. This will be much like any other nondemand genital caress, where one partner is active and the other is passive. As with any sensate focus exercise, exchange focusing caresses.

The Exercise If you are the active partner, pleasure your partner with a front caress and genital caress for about fifteen minutes. When you've finished, say so. If you are the passive partner, experience the sensations, without speaking, unless something is hurting or bothering you. When your partner has finished, you can ask for a repeat of something you liked.

You can ask your partner for a particular type of caress that he or she already did. For example, say, "I really liked when you licked just under the head of my penis. I'd like you to do that again," or, "I liked when you ran your finger slowly up my lips and over my clitoris. Please do that again."

Notice that each communication includes something about what you liked and a straightforward request to repeat it. This teaches you to use personal "I" statements when talking about sexual matters, and it teaches you to be clear and assertive about asking for what you want.

Active Partner, if you are unclear, ask: "Do you mean like this, or like *this?*" If you're agreeable, spend a few minutes touching your partner in the way he or she likes.

Passive Partner, if your partner starts to repeat something that is not exactly what you want, communicate this. For example, say, "I want you to do it slower" or faster, or whatever it is. Don't settle for anything that is not what you asked for.

Then ask to be touched in a new way.

Each of you should realize that you are always free to say no if you find the request unappealing or objectionable. You can discuss the reasons for it later. Again, "No" does not mean "Not now, not *ever*." It simply means, "I don't want to do that right now."

As you can surmise, there are other ways to ask for sex that are not as effective. For example, some people don't feel comfortable asserting themselves and so they hedge it by saying, "It would be nice if you touched my penis" or even, "You wouldn't want to touch my penis, would you?"

That type of communication does not work. If you want to receive something from your partner, you need to ask for it in an assertive way: "I would like this," or "I want you to do that." You also need to be very specific about the exact type of caress you want. For example, say, "Please put your finger into my vagina slowly and move it slowly in and out," rather than, "Put your finger inside me."

Pointers for the Passive Partner   There are a couple of pitfalls you can fall into while doing this exercise. One is to spend so much time worrying about what you are going to ask for, that you don't enjoy the genital caress while it is happening. Trust me, you will remember something your partner did that you liked. Try to keep an open mind while receiving the caress and focus on your sensations the way you normally would during any caress. You will also be able to think of something your partner didn't do that you would like to try.

Also, when you are receiving the caress and you ask for something, take some time to allow yourself to enjoy it. Don't decide in two seconds, "Oh, this is not really what I wanted." Give yourself a chance to enjoy it. On the other hand, you might make a snap decision to ask for some other kind of caress a few seconds after the first, and that's okay, too. You are free to ask for whatever you want. Your partner will not think it's strange if you change your mind.

Pointers for the Active Partner There are more and less effective ways to hear what your partner says to you. Let's say your partner asks you to repeat a particular type of touch by saying, "I liked it when you caressed my scrotum. Please do that again for a few minutes."

The less effective way to interpret this would be, "Of all the things I did, that was the only thing he liked?" or, "Are you sure you want that? Why not something else?" Try not to read too much into a simple request if you can help it.

It also doesn't help if you wonder, "Why didn't I think of that?" Instead, realize that your partner is sharing with you by telling you something about what he or she wants and likes *right now*.

One more caution: because you know your partner wants something and has asked for it, you may forget to do the caressing for your own pleasure and fall back into "pleasing" your partner. This is probably the toughest thing about adding communication to the nonverbal exercises you have done before. You have to develop a mindset in which you are able to touch for your own pleasure, even though you know that your partner is enjoying it, too. If you are able to strike this balance between pleasing yourself and being consciously aware that you are pleasing your partner, you have reached the state we call *mutuality*—a sense that you and your partner are sharing a deeply pleasurable experience.

Observe, Reflect, Ask

This is a basic communication exercise that can be adapted for use during sexual activity. It is especially helpful for those of you who have a difficult time saying anything during sex. Many people who are uncommunicative are this way because they are shy or self-conscious, not because they are withdrawn or antisocial. If your partner is prone to complain, "I never know what you like," then this one's for you. You may even find it *stimulating* to ask for what you want sexually.

The Exercise   Start with focusing caresses. As before, decide who will be the active partner first.

Active Partner   Pleasure your partner with a front caress, genital caress, and oral sex. Enjoy this sensual loving for about twenty minutes.

Passive Partner   In this exercise, you won't wait until the end to say what you like and what you don't like. Instead, stop your partner at some point into the exercise when there is something you really like going on. First, think to yourself: "My partner is stroking my penis in a way I particularly like." This is the **observe** phase. Then repeat that same sentence to your partner using an "I" statement: "I like the way you are caressing my penis." This is the **reflect** phase. Then ask your partner to keep doing the caress: "Please caress my penis this way for a few more minutes." This is the **ask** phase. Repeat this process several times during the twenty-minute exercise.

Switch Focus

This exercise can be lots of fun. It calls upon all of your powers of focus and your ability to work harmoniously with each other. I call this "switching focus." It will help you fine-tune your sensate focus abilities, so you can take even more in, and increase feelings of mutuality.

Up to now I have asked you to focus on the exact point of contact between your skin and your partner's skin. But it is possible to focus on touch more specifically. Here are some examples.

If you were doing a genital caress by yourself, you could focus on how your hand felt touching your genitals, or you could focus on how your genitals felt being touched by your hand. You could practice switching your focus back and forth between these two things.

When you are having sexual intercourse, there is a lot more going on than just the sensations in your genitals. You can focus on your own genitals or on your partner's. You can focus on the sensations in other parts of your body. There are also sights, sounds, and smells you can focus on. You are not limited to focusing on just your genitals.

Let me make an analogy to a symphony orchestra. If it is the first time you have ever listened to that type of music, you probably experience it all as one combined sound. But with a little more experience, you can pay attention to the different sections—strings, woodwinds, et cetera. If you have experience playing a musical instrument yourself, you may even be able to pick out the sounds of the individual instruments.

The same idea applies to sexual activity. The more experience you have, the finer the sensations you will be able to focus on. Let's start with the simplest version of this exercise first.

The Exercise Begin this exercise with focusing caresses, then lie in a comfortable side-by-side position in which you can touch each other's genitals with one hand.

Caress each other's genitals simultaneously throughout the rest of this exercise. When you begin this mutual caress, both of you should focus on the penis. Then, after several minutes, switch your focus to the woman's genitals. For the next switch, you both concentrate on the man's hand. Switch again and focus on the woman's hand. Remember to breathe and stay relaxed during this exercise.

This is not easy! It really takes concentration to be able to switch your focus to these different aspects of the experience. The easiest way to do the exercise is to put one person in charge of deciding when to make the switch. That person should say, "Now, we'll both focus on your penis," or, "Now, we'll both focus on my hand."

Taking the Exercise Further   After you have practiced switching your focus back and forth among single items, try focusing on more than one source of sensations as once. For example, practice focusing on both the woman's hand and the man's penis. Or practice focusing on both of your hands at the same time. Then try to focus on the combined sensations. Again, you may find this easier if one partner takes charge of deciding what to focus on and for how long. You can take turns at this if you like.

Switching focus is a skill that can definitely increase your feelings of mutuality, since you know that both you and your partner are concentrating on very specific sensations at the same time. You can use these switch focus skills in any sexual activity—oral sex, intercourse, and especially mutual oral sex, the classic "sixty-nine" position.

Once you know how to do the basic switch focus technique, you can practice different versions of this exercise. Try one version in which one partner is active with oral sex. The active person should practice switching back and forth between how the mouth feels and how the genitals feel in the mouth. This can literally double your enjoyment of oral sex. The passive partner can switch focus between his or her own genitals and how the partner's mouth feels on the genitals. Then switch roles, so you both get practice with all aspects of the exercise. In an exercise like this, it would probably be best for each partner to be in charge of when they switch, as you will both be focusing on different things.

You can also practice switching focus during intercourse. Practice switching back and forth between focusing on the penis and focusing on the vagina. Try this with the woman on her back and the man kneeling between her legs. In this version of the exercise, one person can decide when you will both switch, because you will both focus on the same thing at the same time.

This exercise even makes mutual oral sex better. A lot of people enjoy mutual oral sex, but some find it frustrating. Sometimes, just as you get aroused from your partner's oral caresses, you all of a sudden lose your focus because you're caressing, too—and your arousal level goes down! Practicing the switch focus technique will help *you* control what you focus on and stay with it long enough to remain aroused.

Ask for What You Want

This exercise brings together all of the communication and mutuality skills you have learned in this chapter. It will give you practice at recognizing what you want, asking for it, enjoying it, and switching focus.

This exercise begins the minute you enter the room—you do not do focusing caresses to prepare for it. One person will be active for the first half hour and the other person will be active for the second half hour.

The Exercise   The partner who is active first begins by asking for anything that he or she wants. Let's assume that the woman is active first. Nothing can happen until she requests it. If she wants her partner to remove his clothes, she must say, "Please take off your clothes."

When you are active, you need to tell your partner everything you want him or her to do. You may ask for anything you can think of that you would like your partner to do, but you need to be specific (as you learned to do in the exercise in which you first gave verbal feedback).

If what he does is not exactly what you want, give him directions until he is doing exactly what you want. Feel free to enjoy, for as long as you want, whatever you have asked your partner to do.

When active, you may also do whatever you like, as long as you tell your partner what you are going to do. For example, if you would like to be the initiator for a while, you could say, "I want you to lie back so I can caress your back for a while."

When you are the passive partner, do as your partner asks, unless your partner asks you to do something unpleasant. If that is the case, say, "I don't want to do that right now." There is no need to get into a heavy discussion about why you might not feel like doing a particular activity—you can discuss it later. Your partner will move on and ask for something else.

When you are the passive partner, see if you can do what your partner asks you to. Just remember to approach it in a sensate focus way so that you do it for your own pleasure. See if you can reach that state of mutuality in which you are doing a caress so it feels good to you, but you are aware that your partner is enjoying it too.

When you are in the active role, try not to second-guess your partner. Ask for something *you* want, rather than what you think your partner wants to do.

A secret to success with this exercise is to take a minute to think about what you want, based on your feelings *right now*. Do you feel like doing something to your partner's body, or are you so stressed out that you want your partner to take care of you in some way? Do you feel like doing relaxing and sensual activities, or do you feel like you want something sexual right away?

Whether you are active or passive with this exercise, re-member to focus on your feelings, breathe, and relax. When you are asked to touch your partner in a certain way, touch for your own pleasure, and practice switching your focus back and forth between how your body feels when it is touching, and how your partner's body feels as you touch it.

This is one of the most complicated exercises you can do, in the sense that if you are the passive partner, you practice focusing even though you don't know what your partner will ask for next. But it can be very rewarding.

Stream of Consciousness, Solo

What does a literary technique have in common with your sex life? You can use a stream of consciousness or free association technique to help loosen up your way of communicating with your partner sexually.

Some people feel inhibited about communicating during sex. They censor their thoughts so much that they are no longer capable of purely spontaneous communication. This exercise can help you feel comfortable with free and spontaneous sexual communication.

Do a genital caress by yourself. As you caress yourself, say whatever comes to your mind. Say it out loud, without censoring anything. Because this is uncensored, there is no way to predict what you will say. Your stream could consist of random thoughts, grunts, moans, descriptions of what you are feeling or what is happening, or descriptions of fantasies. You may latch onto one thought and stick with it, or jump from one meaningless phrase to other.

The first time you do this exercise, you will be very self-conscious. If you spend fifteen minutes at it, you may be lucky to produce twenty seconds of truly uncensored speech. Try to keep talking constantly throughout the exercise, even if what you say sounds silly or doesn't make sense. That's the whole point. If you are having difficulty, you can always fall back on *describing* what you are feeling. This is a way of communicating that is most likely to be uncensored. If you do this exercise by yourself a few times, it can loosen you up so that it will be easier to have spontaneous communication when you are with your lover.

Stream of Consciousness, Together

Now I'd like you to use this exercise to develop trust between you and your lover.

Lie on your back and have your partner caress your genitals. As your partner caresses you, say whatever comes to your mind without censoring or editing. Just the experience of receiving a genital caress will help bring spontaneous sexual thoughts to the surface. This is unconscious material and may include emo-tional nonverbal communication such as moaning or crying.

If you are caressing your partner during this exercise, con-centrate on caressing in a way that feels best to you. Don't even pay attention to what your partner is saying. Just gently remind him or her to keep talking if the verbal stream stops. The caressing partner could even wear earphones at first to make the verbal partner less self-conscious. This exercise can help you share an intimate emotional experience with your partner as you bring up a lot of unconscious material.

When you've finished, find a mutually agreeable way to bring this exercise to a close. You may need to talk with each other about what came up, or you may feel so sexually charged you choose to make love. If you need comforting after this exercise, use one of the bonding positions I described at the beginning of the chapter. Do whatever feels natural.

If this exercise got a little "heavy" for you, light relief is on the way. See if the following suggestions don't bring a new sense of youthful exuberance to your physical relationship.

Remembering to Play

Most of the sensate focus exercises you have done so far have been fairly structured. It's a good idea to let loose every once in a while and just play. As Aphra Ben wrote, "Variety is the soul of pleasure."

In that spirit, I'd like to offer you some playful, sensual activities you can enjoy together. Allow them to inspire you to create your own ways to play together. The spontaneity of play makes sex all the more fresh.

The Foot Caress

The foot caress includes a foot bath and it is very relaxing. Since it only involves the ankles and feet, you can even do it clothed, if you like. I usually bathe each foot for about five minutes and caress each foot with lotion for about five minutes. This exercise can stimulate sexual desire because it is so relaxing. Use it if your partner has had a bad day and needs some deep relaxation to feel ready for sex.

Before you begin, gather two towels, a basin large enough for a person's feet, liquid soap, lotion, hot water, and a comfortable chair for the person whose feet are being washed.

Active Partner Fill the basin with warm water and place your partner's feet in the water. Add the liquid soap and slowly caress your partner's feet in the water. Caress as you would for any other sensate focus exercise, touching for your own pleasure. Don't massage the feet but rather, keep the touch slow and light. Bathe one foot at a time.

When you are done with both feet, lift one foot at a time, dry the feet, and wrap them in separate towels. Then take one foot from a towel and caress it using the lotion.

Passive Partner   The only thing you need to do is relax and enjoy. Allow yourself to feel pampered. Relax your feet and legs. You don't even have to lift your feet to put them in the basin—your partner will do it.

The Sensuous Shower

The sensuous shower is a whole-body caress that takes place in the shower. The purpose is not to soap up and get clean, but to enjoy your body and your lover's body along with the added sensation of water.

There are a number of ways to do this. Just taking a shower together is a good bonding exercise for some couples. You can also practice any of the sensate focus caresses, with each of you taking a turn at being the active partner. Or, simply make the caresses mutual.

Use liquid soap and caress any part of your partner's body that feels good. Caress for your own pleasure when you are active.

If you become aroused during the sensuous shower, just enjoy the feelings of your partner caressing you and the water beating down on your skin. If you have an erection, an orgasm, or an ejaculation, enjoy them. Some people like to have intercourse in the shower standing up. Just be careful because some types of soap can irritate the penis and vagina.

The Tom Jones Dinner

Sensuality includes all five senses, not just touch. And sensuality isn't just sexual.

In the Tom Jones dinner, named for the sensuous eating

scene from the movie, you prepare several foods that can be eaten with the hands. There are three rules—no feeding yourself, no talking, and no utensils. This exercise will help you get into the purely sensuous aspects of eating, free from the restraint of table manners.

First, choose appropriate foods. Some suggestions are: fruit (especially juicy ones such as oranges and peaches), hors d'oeuvres such as cheese and crackers, any meat that can be pulled off a bone, and anything messy that can be licked off fingers or elsewhere. Things that are creamy or juicy feel especially good in the mouth. For beverages, use wine or champagne if you drink alcohol, or sparkling water or fruit juice if you don't.

Arrange the food on an old sheet to protect your carpeting and furniture. Take off your clothes. Relax, caress each other if you need a transition, then start feeding each other. Eat with the goal of feeling every sensation as the food passes through your lips and moves in your mouth.

Watch your partner eat. Put food on your partner's body and slowly lick it off. If you want a drink, your partner can take the drink and then transfer it to your mouth while kissing.

For fun, arrange the foods into the shapes of genitals, breasts and buttocks, and watch your partner lick and eat them. Feel free to belch and make lip-smacking noises and all of those other things you're not supposed to do in polite society. If you spill some food on yourself, don't worry about it. You can lick it off, or better yet, your partner can lick it off. Finish the Tom Jones dinner by washing each other off with warm wet towels, or by taking a sensuous shower.

Exciting the Five Senses

This ones requires a little thought. You'll need to gather together just the right combination of elements to engage all five of your partner's senses. Each of you can take turns at being the bearer of delights.

When it's your turn to prepare the room, for example, you might choose to light a jasmine-scented candle to appeal to your lover's sense of smell, wear something sexy that's pleasing to the eyes, and play some soulful music on the stereo. Then you might uncork your lover's favorite wine to stimulate the taste buds, and use your fingertips or palms to caress his or her skin.

This allows you to combine a sensate focus exercise with the sensual pleasures you know your partner likes.

When it's your turn to be passive, allow yourself to focus on each of the different senses. One stimulus for each sense is plenty. If there are too many things going on in a room, it is distracting.

Body Decoration

Body paints can also give you hours of fun. Some are even edible. You can buy these at an adult store or through a catalog.

Try this in the bathtub or shower, or some private grove outside. If you decide to paint each other indoors, protect your furniture and carpets with plastic.

Be outlandish with your designs. The more primitive, the better. Use this as a gateway into the more animal, primal aspect of sexuality. Moan, growl, and lightly chew on your partner. Make love while still decorated. If the paints are edible, you can lick them off each other. Try playing some tribal music to help you get into the spirit of this.

Mutual Orgasm

Timing your orgasm so that you come at the same moment, while you gaze into each other's eyes, requires an openness and an ability to be at one with each other as you make love. Practice this union with a sense of celebration of all that you learned since you experienced your first sensate focus session.

This exercise takes you back to the basics—focusing, breathing, and relaxing. It allows you to combine things that you like about your previous style of lovemaking with the sensate focus techniques you have learned in this book. Notice how sensate focus changes your lovemaking.

Before You Begin   Start with some unstructured foreplay—anything you and your lover like to do to prepare for making love. Decide on a position for intercourse in advance, and use any one where you and your lover are face to face.

The Exercise   In this more advanced version of nondemand penetration, the partner who is on top controls the speed of the thrusting, and should start as slowly as possible. The other partner should follow at the same speed. Both should focus on the sensations arising out of the contact between the penis and the vagina. Relax and breathe.

Men, think of yourself as caressing the inside of your lover's vagina with your penis.

Women, think of yourself as caressing your lover's penis with the walls of your vagina.

Look at each other as you move. Keep your muscles as relaxed as possible and remember to breathe. If you've done the many peaking exercises earlier in the book, your awareness of your arousal levels is probably automatic for you now. You probably also have a good idea of how aroused your partner is. The best cues for that are heart rate and breathing.

When the person on top reaches the beginning of orgasm,

the other should follow. As you reach orgasm, take a deep breath, relax your body, open your eyes wide, and look deep into your partner's eyes.

Mutual orgasm is an amazing feeling and once you've had the experience together, you may think that this is as good as sex gets. Believe it or not, there are levels of sexual experience that go beyond even this. I call them healing and ecstasy, and I discuss them in the next chapter.

Chapter Thirteen

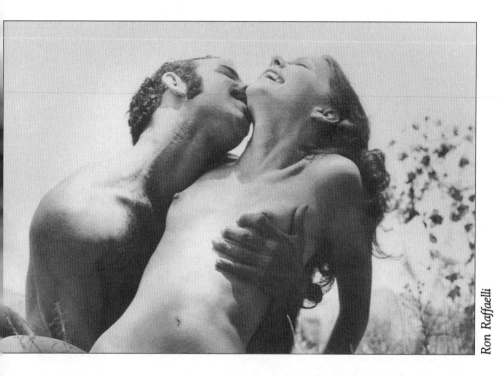

Ron Raffaelli

Beyond Sensate Focus—
Sexual Healing and Ecstacy

I 'll bet a funny thing happens on the road to making love better and better—you wake up one morning and notice that your skin is glowing, and that you and your beloved are radiating well-being.

Regular practice of the sensate focus techniques can do this. And much more.

As you've no doubt experienced, sensate focus is *very* relaxing. If you are able to set aside time for one to three sessions per week, you may even notice that your body becomes conditioned to this level of relaxation and more resistant to physical and psychological stress.

The sensate focus program provides you with regular exposure to the healing power of touch. We talked about how essential touch is to good health back in Chapter 2.

These exercises provide your brain with the stimulation of learning something new—which can bring a rejuvenating freshness back into the rest of your life.

And of course, they provide you with ample doses of life-affirming, physical pleasure. You may find that you feel more at home in your body than ever. After all, your body is the source of that wonderful pleasure.

These sensate focus exercises also help you and your partner strengthen your love for each other, as you learn to communicate better, build trust, and become more and more intimate. Research shows that a loving relationship to a committed partner is perhaps the single, strongest psychological predictor of resistance to illness and premature death.

Clearly, the time you spend practicing these exercises brings benefits above and beyond becoming better lovers. I know from watching my clients that the gains spill over into other areas of life.

Did you know, for instance, that this kind of pressure-free sexual activity is one of the best treatments for stress, anxiety, and depression? A healthy, satisfying sexual relationship can also increase your confidence and build your self-esteem. I have seen client's lives transformed as they became more comfortable about their sexuality and more confident about themselves. The sexual energy in our bodies is so basic it enlivens everything about us when given the space for full expression.

Making love is just as regenerative for the body. Research has shown that it can help boost immunity, improve cardiovascular fitness, lessen premenstrual syndrome, and dissolve aches and pains. This is because sexual activity helps you release endorphins, the body's natural painkillers.

Learning the sensate focus exercises together can even heal a troubled relationship. You simply can't do them well unless you learn to shut out the world temporarily and concentrate totally on each other. Gradually, you get into the habit of setting aside time to be with each other in a pleasurable way, and to communicate honestly about your needs and feelings. Research shows that people who know how to communicate their feelings, in both verbal and nonverbal ways, are healthier—both physically and emotionally.

You can learn to intensify the healing power of sex by consciously focusing it when you make love. Some esoteric eastern traditions even prescribe certain positions and sexual exercises to heal specific organs. While that is beyond the scope of this book, I would like to teach you a simple way to experience the healing power of sex.

Sexual Healing

There is little that can do more to boost your sense of well-being than knowing that your partner cares for you and desires you sexually. One way to express this to each other is to take turns making love to each other. Do it in a way that allows you to give yourself 100 percent to the experience.

Have your partner lie back and relax. Lovingly lock your gaze on your partner's eyes as you psychologically draw your partner in and compel him or her to focus on what you are doing. The more you enjoy what you're doing, and the more intently you focus, the more effective this will be.

Caress your partner's body with your hands. Place your ear on top of your partner's chest so you can hear his or her heartbeat. Maintain as much body contact as you can. As you start to caress your partner's genitals, keep your ear or a hand on his or her heart. Or keep your face up against your partner's face. Maintain this contact as you begin to have slow, gentle, focused intercourse with your partner.

As you make love, concentrate all your mental energy toward healing or nurturing your partner psychologically. This is a lot different than worrying about whether your partner likes what you are doing. Here, you are directing all of your positive sexual energy toward making your lover feel good, rather than trying to make your lover feel good *about you* because you are using the "right" technique or touching in the "right" place.

If you both make love with the intention to focus your innate healing abilities on each other, this can be very powerful. You might even feel the healing energy that you have created together as an intensified current between you. This type of union is intensely fullfilling. Yet, you can have an even deeper experience of sexual communion. It's called ecstasy.

Ecstasy

Ecstatic sex is a level of sexual experience beyond arousal, beyond the intense pleasure of orgasm, and even beyond mutuality and intimacy. It comes unbidden during intercourse, and most typically, just at the point of orgasm. There is no mistaking it when it happens.

You and your partner may feel yourselves becoming so close that you merge into one, transcending the limits of your bodies. Or, you alone may feel the bliss shooting up your spine and catapulting you into a dimension of experience you can only describe as cosmic.

I have experienced it myself and it is hard to put into words.

I've found it most like those descriptions of the Buddhist state of being totally free from desire. It is a state of pleasure so intense, that while it may be accompanied by an orgasm, you really don't know whether you're having an orgasm or not. And you both turn to each other and say, "Did you feel *that?* What *was* that?"

Spiritual experiences are so highly personal, that I cannot describe a typical ecstatic moment. But here are ways my clients have described it:

"While my husband and I were having sex, I had several orgasms in a row, and then I just seemed to stay in this orgasmic state. I felt like I was there for several minutes although it couldn't have been more than a few seconds. My husband told me my eyes glazed over. It was like being in an altered state of consciousness."

"I saw God, Buddha, and Allah." (Yes, he was being metaphorical.)

"When I got close to orgasm, I felt this white-hot light start at my tailbone and slowly move up my spine. When it got to my head, I had the orgasm. It was one of the strangest things I've ever felt. I asked my wife if she felt anything strange and she said she felt almost like both of us lifted about six inches off the bed."

Some people have said that they see intense colors or images. Others hear music. Some feel an overwhelming sense of connection with all creation. These experiences are probably due in part to the release of endorphins—besides killing pain, endorphins can cause intensely pleasurable states.

Ecstatic sex is something you cannot make happen. Every time I've experienced it, it has been unplanned. Yet, I do know that the sensate focus approach is much more likely to lead to ecstatic sex than a performance-oriented approach. This is because the state of mind that is a prerequisite for ecstatic sex demands that you be in the here and now and one hundred percent focused on your sensations.

The ecstasy associated with intense sexual experiences is the focus of a form of yoga known as tantra. Tantric yoga emphasizes reuniting the basic male and female principles in the cosmos through specific practices and postures. The sexual energy is harnessed in a way that can lead the practitioners to transcendence and ecstasy. Tantra can be practiced by both couples and individuals. After you have completed the exercises in *Sexual Pleasure*, you may wish to learn more about tantric yoga or tantric sex in order to go further in your exploration of your sexual self. Margo Anand's book, *The Art of Sexual Ecstasy: The Path of Sacred Sexuality for Western Lovers* is a worthwhile book on this subject.

Going Forward from Here

Through the exercises in this book, you have learned to enjoy touching and being touched. You have learned to let go—to relax and enjoy your own sexual response, to savor your desire for your partner. Through peaking and plateauing exercises you have also learned to make the most of your arousal and orgasm patterns. And through it all, you have learned to communicate with your partner and become deeply intimate.

Where do you go from here?

I recommend that you continue the breathing, PC-muscle, and bonding exercises daily for the rest of your life. They will keep your senses, your body, and your passion alive and afire.

Return to the others as you need or desire. Remember that you can always count on the focusing caresses to relax you. Since you have learned peaking and plateauing, your body has been conditioned and will naturally respond in that way. This gives you infinite options on ways to make love, based on what you have come to learn about your own sexual responses and possibilities.

Sexual expression can have an overwhelmingly positive effect on your life. It frees you, enriches you, and opens up new dimensions of your humanity. I hope the sensual and sexual activities you have learned here will help you enjoy the many healthy and empowering aspects of sexuality—desire, arousal, orgasm, intimacy, and possibly ecstasy.

Appendix A
Male and Female
Sexual Anatomy

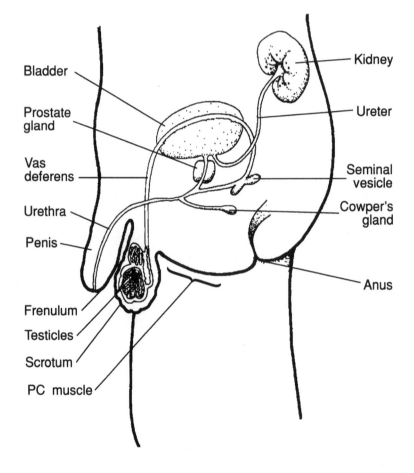

Bladder

Prostate gland

Vas deferens

Urethra

Penis

Frenulum

Testicles

Scrotum

PC muscle

Kidney

Ureter

Seminal vesicle

Cowper's gland

Anus

Male Sexual Anatomy

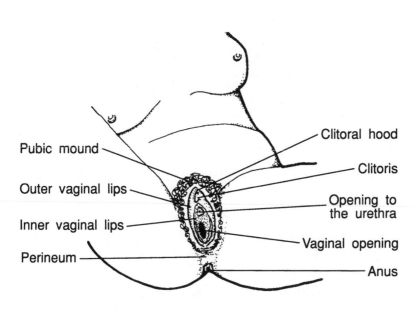

Pubic mound

Outer vaginal lips

Inner vaginal lips

Perineum

Clitoral hood

Clitoris

Opening to the urethra

Vaginal opening

Anus

External Female Sexual Anatomy

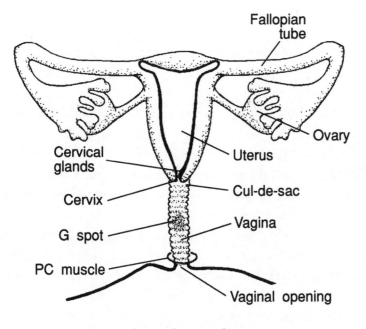

Fallopian tube

Cervical glands

Cervix

G spot

PC muscle

Ovary

Uterus

Cul-de-sac

Vagina

Vaginal opening

Internal Female Sexual Anatomy

Appendix B
Help for Common Problems

At some point in his or her sexual life, almost everybody faces a performance difficulty or questions their orgasmic capabilities. If you have had specific concerns or problems with your sexual functioning, the sensate focus exercises in this book will not only work for you, they can *help* you overcome these difficulties. This section addresses some common concerns for men (such as rapid ejaculation) and for women (such as inability to orgasm during intercourse). They offer exercises or modifications that will make the exercises in this book more successful and more fulfilling for you.

Erections

If you have had problems with erections in the past, you can still use the exercises in Chapter 7. Start by determining whether your erection problems are physical or psychological.

If you have not had early morning or nighttime erections in some time, or if you never have erections with masturbation, your erection problems may be physical. In that case, you will need to consult a urologist who specializes in erection problems. As I mentioned in Chapter 6, there are a number of physical problems that can affect your erections.

On the other hand, if you have erections when you wake up in the morning, but not with your lover, it is likely that your erection problems are psychological; you will benefit greatly from the exercises described Chapter 7.

Before you do the exercises in Chapter 7, try the following

"Nondemand Penetration" exercise. It has helped many men work through their anxiety about erections. Remember to take your time and to do them with a partner you feel secure with. Go slowly, repeat the exercise if you need to, and *focus, breathe, and relax*.

Nondemand Penetration

Many men with erection problems are able to have erections with oral stimulation, but have performance anxiety when they attempt intercourse. This exercise can help to overcome that. It can be used when you reach the point that you are able to have erections with oral sex and peaking.

Before You Begin   Start with focusing caresses and then do a nondemand front caress or genital caress with your partner.

The Exercise   Lie on your back and have your partner start your peaking process with her hands and tongue. If she feels you are maintaining an erection, she can get on top of your penis and have intercourse for a few strokes. You should stay totally passive. There is no demand on you to maintain your erection or have an ejaculation.

Your partner will do a few strokes of intercourse and then return to the manual and oral peaking.

Have her repeat the nondemand intercourse with more and more strokes each time until you are comfortable and relaxed enough to move without putting pressure on yourself to maintain the erection.

Once you are comfortable with this exercise, you can try some of the erection exercises described in Chapter 7.

Rapid Ejaculation

The exercises described in Chapter 6 can help any man who would like to last longer and prolong his arousal and pleasure during intercourse or other sensual stimulation. Sometimes, though, men may ejaculate so rapidly that they don't have time to enjoy any stimulation at all. If this has been a concern for you at any time, you can still use these exercises, adding the following suggestions:

- Try doing extra PC muscle exercises to moderate your arousal.

- You may find it helpful to repeat the basic exercises a number of times, so that you become more relaxed each time you do them. Don't focus on holding back ejaculation, focus on the sensations.

- It may also be helpful to break some of the exercises into smaller parts. With the peaking exercises, try peaking at levels 1 to 7 in one exercise and then take it higher in the next exercise. If the exercise calls for manual and oral stimulation *and* penetration, wait to do the penetration part in the next session. If the exercise includes two penetration positions, do only one position.

- Have patience with yourself as you learn the 1 to 10 arousal scale.

Finally, don't try to control your ejaculation during any exercise. Relax, breathe, and focus on your sensations. Your body will learn control. Give yourself permission to enjoy ejaculation *whenever* it happens. This will reduce the pressure you may feel and allow your body to reestablish itself. Trust the process—it works.

Difficulties with Ejaculation

Ejaculation is a reflex and you can't *make* it happen. All you can do is relax your PC muscle and allow yourself to try to receive as much stimulation as possible. Concentrate on how good the sensuous contact feels rather than worrying about whether or not you will ejaculate.

If you have any difficulty ejaculating, the exercises in Chapter 6 and the penile sensitivity exercises in Chapter 8 will help you. What you have to watch out for is a tendency to *work* at ejaculating. If you are having intercourse and you realize that you are working at trying to ejaculate, you need to stop and back up to an earlier exercise, or at least an earlier stage of the exercise, where you feel relaxed. You may have to set a time limit for yourself for intercourse and just stop at fifteen or twenty minutes whether you are close to ejaculation or not. Remember that you are doing these exercises to enhance your *pleasure*, rather than pressure yourself to perform.

Some men are able to ejaculate easily with masturbation or oral stimulation, but have difficulty ejaculating with intercourse or do not have as strong an ejaculation. The exercises in those chapters, along with the following two, can help you develop stronger ejaculations with intercourse.

Changing Positions for Men

If you get into the habit of masturbating in only one position you may find that's the only position you can ejaculate in. If you vary your masturbation position, it will help you ejaculate more easily in different positions during intercourse.

A good way to do this is to practice the peaking process by yourself described in Chapter 3. Do one peak in your preferred position, say on your back, and then another peak in a new position, like kneeling or lying on your side. Alternate positions until you are able to peak up to an 8 or 9 in a new position.

Then peak up almost to the point of inevitability in your preferred position. At the instant before you ejaculate, roll over into the new position so that you reinforce ejaculation and orgasm in the new position. After a few sessions practicing these new positions, you will be able to masturbate all the way to ejaculation in a position different than the one you have used for years. This ability will help tremendously when you have intercourse with your partner.

Ejaculating with Intercourse

Do the whole peaking and plateauing progression I described in Chapter 8, to see what level of arousal you can easily reach with intercourse. Let's say that you can comfortably reach a level 8 with intercourse without feeling that you are working at it. At that point withdraw from your partner's vagina and masturbate until you reach a 9.

Then insert again and peak as high as you can with intercourse. Keep alternating masturbation and intercourse peaks until you wish to ejaculate. Masturbate up to the point of inevitability and insert quickly so that you ejaculate in your partner's vagina.

The toughest thing about this is staying comfortable and not putting pressure on yourself. You may need to rehearse the exercise a few times to find out which masturbation positions and intercourse positions are the easiest, most relaxing, and comfortable for you and your partner.

Female Orgasm

The exercises in Part III, The Female Sexual Pleasure Cycle, can help any woman develop her ability to have powerful orgasms, whether she has had them before or not. But what if you have tried every exercise at least three times and you still have not been able to have an orgasm during intercourse? Don't give up—I have another suggestion: manually stimulate your clitoris during intercourse.

The reason you may not have been able to have an orgasm during intercourse is that the internal orgasm triggers (the G spot, cervix, and cul-de-sac) don't work for you yet. Until they do, your clitoris is your most reliable orgasm trigger. The problem is, many intercourse positions don't stimulate the clitoris enough for you to have an orgasm. If you or your partner manually stimulate your clitoris during intercourse, your chances of having an orgasm will greatly increase.

Sex therapists call this a "bridge maneuver." In behavioral psychology, a bridge maneuver is an activity that connects two behaviors that you already know how to do to form a new behavior. Here the two behaviors you already know how to do are how to have intercourse and how to have an orgasm with masturbation.

The Bridge Maneuver for Women

Begin a session with focusing caresses and then have your partner lie on his back. Do a genital caress and have oral sex with him until he gets an erection.

Climb on top of your partner and begin peaking and plateauing using his penis to pleasure yourself. As you reach high peaks and plateaus (7, 8, and 9), stimulate your clitoris with your fingers and *focus*.

Masturbate to orgasm by stimulating your clitoris *and* allowing your partner's penis to stroke you. Notice the added sensations of simultaneous masturbation and intercourse. With some practice, you will need less and less direct clitoral stimulation with your fingers, and your ability to have an orgasm will transfer to the stimulation of intercourse.

There are two other variations of this exercise. They both work best when you are on top. Ask your partner to stimulate your clitoris with his hand, instead of doing it yourself. Or, either one of you can use a vibrator or dildo to stimulate your clitoris once you have reached a high level of arousal.

If Anxiety Has Been a Concern . . .

You can do the exercises in this book if sexual anxiety has been a problem for you. The only suggestion I have is that you may want to go a little more slowly and break some of the exercises into two or three different parts if you need to. Also, if during any new exercise you recognize that you are anxious and the exercise is not helping, back up to a previous exercise with which you felt more comfortable. Then try the new exercise again at a later time.

It does not do any good to continue an exercise if you have either physical or mental anxiety that won't go away. If you are in the active role and you notice that your partner is not able to relax during an exercise, back up to something with which he or she feels more comfortable. The key to sensual focus is finding out what feels best, at your own pace, with your own pleasure points.

Suggested Reading

The Art of Sexual Ecstasy: The Path of Sacred Sexuality for Western Lovers. Margo Anand. Los Angeles: Jeremy P. Tarcher, Inc., 1989.

Bioenergetics. Alexander Lowen. New York: Penguin Books, 1975.

For Yourself: The Fulfillment of Female Sexuality. Lonnie G. Barbach. New York: Anchor Books, 1975.

Human Sexual Inadequacy. William Masters and Virginia Johnson. Boston: Little, Brown and Company, 1970.

The Perfect Fit: How to Achieve Mutual Fulfillment and Monogamous Passion Through the New Intercourse. Edward Eichel and Phillip Nobile. New York: Donald I. Fine Publishers, 1992.

The Relaxation Response. Herbert Benson. New York: William Morrow and Company, 1975.

Super Potency. Dudley Danoff. New York: Warner Books, 1992.

Touching: The Human Significance of the Skin. Ashley Montagu. New York: Harper & Row, 1986.

Touching for Pleasure: A 12-Step Program for Sexual Enhancement. Adele P. Kennedy and Susan Dean, Ph.D. Chatsworth, CA: Chatsworth Press, 1988.

About the Photographers

Steven Baratz, 37, is a commercial photographer whose work has been exhibited in Massachusetts, New York, and California. He is a graduate of the Art Center College of Design.

Morgan Cowin, 47, is a freelance photographer who has taught photojournalism at the University of Nairobi, and classical guitar at the Kenya Conservatory of Music. His work has been published in *California Loving, Co-Evolution Quarterly, National Geographic World, Cupido,* and *Sierra Magazine.*

"I have always been intrigued by nude bodies. Most of my subjects are not classic beauties (I even have a 92-year-old woman friend whom I long to photograph), but I see something worth celebrating in each of them. Recording their loss of inhibition and their growing freedom to express themselves in an intimate fashion is fascinating to me. I regard the photographic experience as a collaborative effort. I want my subjects to feel good about the end product, and about our time together."

Clytia Fuller, 44, has been a lesbian feminist photographer for over 17 years, with an emphasis on photographing those aspects of women not traditionally shown. She has been published in *WomanSpirit, Plexus, Lesbian Health, Matters, Lesbian Words II, The Blatant Image,* and other feminist publications. She has two children.

Hella Hammid was a freelance photographer for such publications as *Life, Town and Country, Ebony,* and *The New York Times.* She published several books, including *The Sensible Book* and *A is for Aloha,* and photographed such personalities as Benjamin Spock, Edward Weston, Imogen Cunningham, Alexander Lowen, and Anais Nin. Her work has been exhibited in many galleries and museums, and is included in *The Family of Man.*

"My nudes are about ephemera—sensual trigger-points for the imagination."

Ron Raffaelli, 50, is a widely-known producer of erotic still photography and videotapes. His photographs have appeared in various one-man shows, and in a Smithsonian Institute exhibition on American advertising. He has produced album covers and still photographs for the Beatles, the Rolling Stones, Jimi Hendrix, the Doors, the Osmonds, and Liberace. He has published three volumes of erotic photography, *Rapture, Desire,* and *Temptations,* and has produced over 70 erotic films.

"The first time our parents punished us when we were caught in the innocent act of sex-play, a sensual Garden of Eden vanished, which it is the responsibility of the erotic artists to recreate and vivify. The laughter, fondling, licking, and kissing are natural human manifestations, but once abandoned they are difficult to rediscover. The role of the erotic artists must be more than simply to entertain: I must strike an innocent, long-silent chord in the viewer's imagination—that part of us which unabashedly plays with our sexuality, experiments, laughs at our awkwardness, and celebrates every sensuous success."

Ron Turner, 44, has traveled through India, Nepal, and Mexico as an itinerant photographer. He is the founder of Focal Point Gallery and Press. His recent photographic work includes development of the "phototern," a process of bleaching, redeveloping, and painting with photochemicals on a developed and fixed photographic print. He has published one book of photography, *Nudes: 1975–85.*

"The nude has always been an endless source of inspiration for me. Whether seeing the portrait of a body, or exploring the reciprocal properties of line and space, the nude has helped me discover a universal language."

Photographs reprinted from *Erotic by Nature: A Celebration of Life, of Love, and of Our Wonderful Bodies,* David Steinberg, ed. *Erotic by Nature* is a collection of erotic writing and photography for women and men of all ages and lifestyles. Hardbound, 224 oversize pages, 122 duotone photographs, 15 stories, 17 drawings, 38 poems. Available from Red Alder Books, P.O. Box 2992, Santa Cruz CA 95063. $39.50 postpaid, or send a self-addressed, stamped envelope for an illustrated brochure.

Index

EXTENDED MASSIVE ORGASM: How You Can Give and Receive Intense Sexual Pleasure

by Steve Bodansky, Ph.D., & Vera Bodansky, Ph.D.

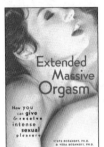

Yes, extended massive orgasms can be achieved! In this hands-on guide, Steve Bodansky and his wife Vera describe how to take the experience of sex to a new level of enjoyment. Focusing primarily on women but addressing the needs of men as well, the authors disclose knowledge that is practically unknown except to specialized researchers and involves the stimulation of specific and uniquely sensitive areas. They recommend the best positions for orgasm and offer strategic advice for every technique from seduction to kissing. No matter how long a couple has been together, it's never too late—or too early—to make each other ecstatic in the bedroom. The Bodanskys explain how.

224 pp. 6 illus. 12 b/w photos ... Paperback $14.95

SIMULTANEOUS ORGASM and Other Joys of Sexual Intimacy *by* Michael Riskin, Ph.D., & Anita Banker-Riskin, M.A.

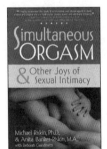

Based on techniques developed at the Human Sexuality Institute, this guide shows couples how they can achieve the special, intimate experience of simultaneous orgasm.

The first part examines research on simultaneous orgasm, the second describes specific techniques and gives step-by-step instructions to help individuals achieve orgasm separately, then simultaneously. Each exercise includes practical advice for relaxing and feeling comfortable with your own sexuality and that of your partner. A separate section explains the purpose of the exercise and offers insights about how it can positively affect your relationship. The authors also explore gender differences and the emotional connections and rewards of achieving simultaneous orgasm.

240 pp. ... 9 b/w photos ... Paperback $14.95 ... Hardcover $24.95